SOAR
INTO HEALTH

Simple Principles to Health and Wellness
Eat Well. Move Well. Sleep Well. Soar On.

Dr. Carolyn Dolan DPT, Cert MDT

authorHOUSE®

AuthorHouse™
1663 Liberty Drive
Bloomington, IN 47403
www.authorhouse.com
Phone: 1 (800) 839-8640

Published by AuthorHouse   01/19/2016

ISBN: 978-1-5049-7277-2 (sc)
ISBN: 978-1-5049-7275-8 (hc)
ISBN: 978-1-5049-7276-5 (e)

Library of Congress Control Number: 2016900460

Print information available on the last page.

This book is printed on acid-free paper.

Source of Photos:
Colin Nicolai Photography
www.cnicphoto.com

CONTENTS

MEDICAL DISCLAIMER

Information in this book is provided for informational purposes only. The information is a result of years of practice experience and research by the author. This information is not intended as a substitute for the advice provided by your physician or other healthcare professional. Do not use this information from this book to treat or diagnose a health problem or disease, or prescribing medication or other treatment. Always speak with your physician or other healthcare professional before taking any medication or nutritional, herbal or homeopathic supplement, or using any treatment for a health problem. If you have or suspect that you have a medical problem, contact your health care provider promptly. Do not disregard professional medical advice or delay in seeking professional advice because of something you have read in this book. Information provided in this book does not create a healthcare provider-patient relationship between you and the author. Information and statements regarding dietary supplements have not been evaluated by the Food and Drug Administration and are not intended to diagnose, treat, cure, or prevent any disease.

ABOUT THE BOOK

This book is part memoir, part story, and part self-help. It is the sharing of information and experiences that may help others to improve their health status, treat their patients, and even raise their family. It is a synthesis of many research articles in the field of health, rehabilitation, medicine, nutrition, sleep, and much more in a useable and clear format that everyone can understand. Achieving health and wellness while reducing chronic disease is the goal of *Soar Into Health*.

DEDICATION

To my husband and three children:
Thank you for teaching me more about myself than I ever thought
I needed to know. You are the reasons why I do what I do.

Dear Ryan, Keenan, and Allison,

You are what drive me to be the best mother I can be. As you grow, I am continually challenged as your needs from me change. I worry that it is happening too fast. I worry that I may forget to share any lessons or knowledge that I have gained over the years with you before you leave our home and continue to become the best you that you can be.

I have read, researched, and experienced many things in my life. So has your father. Your father has a steel trap of a memory, but I do not. So I have to have reference material to jog my memory. I have rewatched movies years later and gotten halfway through before I remembered I had watched this movie before. Your father remembers events well. I joke that he has a lot of useless details in there, but it allows him to connect with almost anyone. Then there is me with my nominal aphasia and problems with name retrieval, yet I can remember their backstories, like how they injured themselves or how many kids they have, etc. I hope it is just my brain cleaning up and not signs of early dementia, but either way, it has helped me to write things down.

I may forget something. I won't forget to make you dinner, but the other details may get lost or deemed unimportant for whatever my current reality is. I even started to collect books for you to read before you leave the home and your father's and my influence becomes only a memory. As the world changes for good or bad or simply not fast enough, I want to send you off with maybe just one book to read. Maybe it will also help me remember all those things I have actually learned when life gets busy and I get distracted.

I will try to teach you as best I can, but I know that I am really better at mothering you than I am at directly teaching you. But I love you enough to write this for the future.

It is merely a suggestion. Your life is your own, and you must go on your own journey. I would regret every day if I didn't give you a foundation to help you stand strong when others are doing something different. The reality is that we do things differently than most. Things are changing, and I hope they change quickly, but that may be too optimistic.

The beautiful thing is that you will *always* have a *choice*. And I will always encourage you to respect the opinions of others (including mine, doctors, authority figures) but make your own *informed* decisions. I hope you never take your health for granted. It is a blessing beyond all blessings.

I am honored to be your mother, and I hope that this book helps you when you need it most.

Love,
Mom

Soar (verb)
 a. Fly or rise high in the air
 b. Increase rapidly above the usual level[1]

INTRODUCTION

Nothing in the world is worth having or worth doing unless it means effort, pain, difficulty ... I have never in my life envied a human being who led an easy life. I have envied a great many people who led difficult lives and led them well.

—Theodore Roosevelt

As a traditionally trained physical therapist, I am always seeking to provide simple explanations for patients so that they can easily perform their home-exercise program to recover from injury, illness, or surgery. It sounds easy, but as any health care provider knows, translating what is said or done in the office is often entirely different out of the office. You must translate technical verbiage to layman's terms that the patient will understand. For example, "external rotation of the glenohumeral joint" is meaningless for most. Translating that to "outward rotation of the shoulder" improves the odds of performing the exercise properly, not perfectly, but better. A photo or picture also helps. Proper communication is essential and often difficult.

In the rehabilitation world, we also need to communicate between health care providers, so everyone understands what is going on. Writing every single word and account of everything can be very time-consuming. One way to make it more efficient is to use acronyms. *Acronym*, a noun, is defined by Webster's dictionary as "a word formed from the first (or first few) letters of a series of words, as *radar*, from *ra*dio *d*etecting *a*nd *r*anging." [1] *H*ome *e*xercise *p*rogram becomes HEP. *I*ndependent with *a*ctivities of *d*aily *l*iving becomes IADL. Acronyms commonly are used for procedures in orthopedics, for example, THR—*t*otal *h*ip *r*eplacement, or TKR—*t*otal *k*nee *r*eplacement. These acronyms are very useful in communicating between health care providers and abbreviating to save some time. With the advent of computer documentation, these acronyms aren't nearly as common, and as it turns out, they weren't as clear for communication as they may have been intended.

I am married to an orthopedic surgeon, and my father was an ear, nose, and throat surgeon who had a stint in the military, so I have heard a few other interesting acronyms. A couple of my favorites are military in origin but are often used in the trauma bay. They contain profanity, so I apologize ahead of time, given my initial goal was to make this book family friendly. However, sometimes profanity really gets the message across well, if you know what I mean.

SNAFU—*s*ituation *n*ormal: *a*ll *f*ucked *u*p
FUBAR—*f*ucked *u*p *b*eyond *a*ll *r*ecognition

These may be my favorite. In the past few years during my journey to health, I see these two acronyms daily. We, most humans, have made our lives so complicated that they don't even look like lives anymore. And it has become *normal*. That is the crazy part—that we have become so "fucked up" that we actually believe it is normal.

What I have begun to realize is that our health and wellness should *not* look like immobility and illness, despite how common (or normal) it is today. Even as health care providers, we think it is normal because it is all that we see. Even with our best intentions, we are totally missing the mark. Health care has become solely a *management* system, rather than a *prevention* and *recovery* system. And until a few years ago, I thought that was normal too.

So, as I raise my children and try to care for patients, how do I share the message in an understandable form that my children, patients, and other health care providers will remember what to do and how to apply to their own lives? And that is where another acronym comes to play. It happens to also have a background in the US Navy in 1960 from an engineer at Lockheed Skunk Works:

KISS—*keep it straightforward, stupid,* or *keep it simple, stupid*

I don't mean to imply that anyone specifically is actually stupid. Yet maybe we all are, including me. *Seriously.* Aren't we all just a bit "stupid" to accept being "fucked up" as normal? I know some very smart and intelligent people who accept being "fucked up" as just a normal part of aging and life. I included myself in that group until recently. (Profanity will end from this point on.)

Yet KISS principles, simple principles, can help guide us to health and potentially prevent disease. They may not always be the easiest to do, but they are simple and straightforward when you step back from the craziness and look. It's funny, because my husband, the orthopedic surgeon, said to me once, "Healthy marriage requires that we *kiss* for a whole ten seconds to make a connection." Turns out he made it up. That's ok. I like what it stands for. KISS principles are simple, but not easy. As a healthy kiss requires ten seconds to connect, maybe it takes that long to also make a decision based on KISS principles. Who knows?

One of my favorite quotes is from Theodore Roosevelt. "Nothing in the world is worth having or worth doing unless it means effort." All too often, we fall into habits of convenience and ease, making our lives more complicated and filled with illness. If we had to take a little more time, a little more effort, but could prevent illness and immobility and live our lives full of learning, exploring, connecting, and moving, wouldn't that be worth it? For me, I say absolutely because the results of an "easy and convenient" life scare me to death. Let me explain.

I have seen one too many patients with multiple sclerosis, Parkinson's disease, dementia, Alzheimer's disease, osteoarthritis, rheumatoid arthritis, chronic low-back pain, chronic sprains that fail to recover, and cancer just to name a few. Once you have these diseases, it is hard if not impossible to properly "manage" them and live a life filled with exploring, connecting, movement, or learning. No one deserves these diseases, and by no means are they to blame.

All these years I have tried hard as a physical therapist to help every single patient to the best of my abilities. I can't say that I didn't help most of them, but never did I give them back the lives they used to have. I thought it was my failure. I wasn't a good therapist. I didn't pick the right exercise or do the correct manual treatment. I kept looking for changes on our outcome measures that I saw only change a few points. Only sometimes were there *dramatic* changes. These patients often suffered terribly, especially those with degenerative autoimmune disease like Parkinson's disease or multiple sclerosis. I felt helpless. In the end, it is very egotistical of me to think that I could have done any of that for anyone. What if those patients had known twenty or thirty years ago that eating well, moving well, and sleeping well meant that they would be soaring now? *What if?*

Then one day it changed for my family, my patients, and myself. I discovered the importance of nutrition, the importance of movement, the importance of sleep, and what it means to soar. I didn't discover it all on my own but with lots of reading, research, personal experimentation, and support from my family I discovered something that improved my life. And I have tried to put together KISS principles that will help many. So I write this book in hopes of sharing some of what I have learned. I can't take credit for the information, as many others smarter than all of us already figured it out and continue to share, research, and move health and wellness into today's world. I am merely trying to put it into KISS principles that my children, husband, patients, other health professionals, other mothers, and really anyone can use so they can work on putting KISS principles into their lives to prevent disease, maintain health, and improve their situations. More importantly, I want everyone to be able to make a healthy choice on your own, not dependent on a moneymaking pyramid scheme, not dependent on a health care system that simply *cannot* do it for you.

We are here on this Earth to *soar*, not suffering endlessly without reason or purpose. These few principles will help anyone should they be willing to put in the effort. I hope you start today.

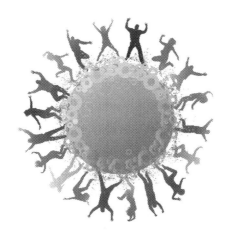

CHAPTER 1: THE BACKSTORY

End range is where the magic happens.

—The McKenzie Institute

As I grew professionally, I continued to keep my personal journey in the background—in part because I didn't think my story was that interesting. I was simply raising three kids and working part-time while my husband started an orthopedic practice in his hometown. We moved a few times, just like everyone else. I really wanted my physical therapy practice to be about the patient, not about me. In the end, maybe my story is meaningful *because* it sounds like everyone else's. I have now realized that we *all* have the same story—just with different details.

I grew up one of three kids in the Bay Area of California. My father was an ear, nose, and throat surgeon. He is officially retired now. My mother is a physical therapist who continues to practice despite being "retired." They were working parents. Growing up, we took regular family vacations, which included frequent exposure to the outdoors and non–city dirt. We also ate steak, potatoes, and salad regularly. We rarely indulged in processed foods. Most of the time, our dessert was homemade blackberry pie made from fruit picked on our property and with butter. I was a healthy and vibrant girl growing up. Like many kids, I had the normal issues; I needed braces because my jaw was too small for my adult teeth. This was probably the first signal of poor nutrition, but it had become so common that no one noticed. I speak more about epigenetics, the study of how external factors influence development, in chapter 2.

Physically, things began to change for me in high school. It wasn't initially dramatic; it seemed like normal teenager stuff: acne, growth spurts, and the like. And even though I wasn't kissing anyone, I even had mononucleosis, the "kissing disease." No one believed me—could you imagine that? I played sports such as basketball, volleyball, tennis, and soccer. I dealt with back pain and getting my period. I struggled with schoolwork and college applications. This doesn't look unusual, yet for a kid who was never sick, feeling pain and dealing with mono were new experiences. When I look back at it now, I was doing mostly okay. I slept well, and as a member of multiple athletic teams, I was getting my exercise. I *appeared* to be thriving because I was getting good grades—but one thing was *dramatically* off: I was not eating real food.

My parents had put me in charge of making my own breakfast and lunch; it's not their fault that I simply didn't eat much. In fact, I can remember buying Cup O' Noodles for lunch and heading to basketball practice after school, none the wiser. Dinners were still mostly healthy thanks to home-cooked meals, but my parents were working. When I was the last kid still at home, "dinner" turned into pizza delivery, Chinese food takeout, or even Kentucky Fried Chicken. Overall, though, I was still doing pretty well.

Then came college. What an amazing experience going off to college was! I lived in the dorms, tried out and ended up playing college basketball, made new friends, and learned a ton. I still slept, but not as well, thanks to all those late-night parties and pizzas to get me through studying. I was still moving well, thanks to time spent riding my bicycle all over campus. I thought I was thriving, but mostly I didn't think about the impact these behaviors had on my health—until I got sick. I almost missed my chemistry final as I lay on my friend's beanbag writhing with abdominal pain. I knew I had to get some help. I was told it was nothing by the student health services. I suspect, in hindsight, this was my start of gluten sensitivity, since I had massive exposure freshman year in college.

I was eating a lot of processed carbs in the form of pizza, pasta, breads, and the like. I was a college athlete, so I had no concerns about weight or anything else, except taking biomedical engineering finals on the road; not many of my teammates were doing that. I struggled mostly with minor injuries from basketball, but in retrospect, I realize that multiple ankle sprains and some intermittent chronic neck/shoulder pain lingered with me for too long. Nothing kept me out of the game much, but the pain was always there.

I kept chugging along and even met Chris, my future husband, in the dorms. We were friends for many years. We enjoyed studying in the library until it closed, playing on intramural basketball teams, and so much more. He even did the color commentary for the campus radio station that covered our basketball games. He was a double major in history and premed, while I was in bioengineering. We were both thriving by the sounds of it—even if we were boring back then.

Once he started medical school, I started physical therapy school in another city. I moved to the city while he stayed at our alma mater. No big deal. Except life was stressful in professional school. I continued similar eating patterns despite my decrease in exercise, and I started cooking more at home, but it still looked like the food I had been eating for years: pizza, pasta, bread, cereal, nonfat milk, and veggies, lots and lots and lots of gluten, refined grains, and sugar. Funny. This looks like the SAD diet, a telling acronym for the standard American diet.

Looking back, that is when two new health challenges emerged: anxiety and toenail fungus. (That may be too much information, but still, it's real life.) Despite the evidence, I brushed it off as normal. Or was this normal? Concerned, I even went to student health services about my toenail fungus. They started me on an oral antifungal medication that is terrible for you in two ways: it attacks your liver, and it is something you shouldn't take if you want to get pregnant. My toenail fungus went away (temporarily, at least). I started counseling for the anxiety. Again, I was learning to be on my own, and that is stressful, right?

I coasted along, finished my master's degree in physical therapy, passed my board exam, and continued on to my doctorate while practicing part-time. We got married before the end of Chris's medical school. Shortly thereafter, as we started our life together, we moved across country to orthopedic residency. It's funny, actually; I swore I would never marry a surgeon, because that is what my dad did. Chris told me when we started dating that he wanted to be either a pediatrician or family practice doc. Those specialties have more regular work hours and shorter residencies. That is not to say that they are easier, but they can be more consistent. Then he did his ortho surgery rotation—and it was all over after that.

When we moved, I was at least realistic about what to expect regarding his time commitment to residency, but I was not prepared for that reality. I was starting to slide down a slippery slope regarding my health, but I did not know it yet. When we started to try to get pregnant, we struggled. Obviously, his work schedule, sleeping habits, and eating were off of what would be considered healthy. Chris had always suffered from strange aches, pains, chronic colds, and severe GERD (gastroesophageal reflux disease), although we didn't have a clear idea of how bad it was until we tried to get pregnant (but that is a story for another book). He also suffered from chronic ear and sinus infections, but that was his standard for most of his life.

When we moved across country, I gained five pounds. Not a big deal, except I remember noticing it and wondering what had happened. I figured it was normal. I was not "fat" by any stretch, but it caught my attention. I had also been on birth control for close to ten years at this point. (I would add that I wish I'd known then what I know now about the effects on my gut microbiome and birth control, but the past is the past. I am all about accepting the past and looking to the future.) We decided to start trying for a baby after his first year at residency, so six months before we started, I stopped taking the birth control pill. We struggled just as many do. As we struggled with fertility for almost a year, we visited obstetricians, got a sperm count, and were just on the verge of seeing a fertility doctor when we finally got pregnant.

In 2006, just before the birth of my first child, I was put on bed rest for gestational hypertension (high blood pressure). The OB was worried about my potential for preeclampsia, a pregnancy condition characterized by high blood pressure that can lead to organ system damage. I remember being home alone once. I had borrowed a blood pressure monitor from a physical therapy colleague of mine so I could assess my blood pressure at home. I had carried laundry from the basement up two flights of stairs, and then I went back down to the main level. (I am bad at bed rest.) After this exertion, I didn't feel well, so I checked my blood pressure. It was 220/160. I checked twice. *Stop everything!* I thought in a panic. *That is a scary number.* As a physical therapist working in the hospital, I check blood pressure all the time. Normal blood pressure should be 120/80. I immediately threw myself down on my left side on the couch and didn't move for about fifteen minutes. When I was ready to recheck my blood pressure, I decided that if things didn't improve, I would call my husband out of the operating room. Fortunately, it resolved down to a safer number. I was lucky I didn't stroke out. Again, this is not abnormal for a first-time pregnancy. I dodged a bullet and ended up delivering a healthy boy with help from forceps, lots of monitors beeping like crazy the whole time, and an epidural that didn't work. Chris, the comedian he is, brought along an "Easy" button from OfficeMax. Do you remember those? The nurses thought he was a jerk, because it was so not easy, but to me, it was funny. So many mothers have stories like this, albeit with different details.

That is when the real fun began. I struggled like crazy with postpartum depression. I struggled with breast-feeding. I struggled getting out of bed. I loved my son, but I simply struggled. I felt like I never produced enough breast milk, and I was exhausted all of the time. I was desperate, but I didn't know what I was desperate for.

I never lost my baby weight altogether, but that was *normal.* Since we struggled for the first pregnancy, we decided to try for number two when it was deemed safe. At the time, we were told nine months. Thinking it would take another year, we tried for number two. My estrogen receptors were primed, and now my body knew how to make a baby, and we got pregnant that first month.

This pregnancy was easier despite my emotional status, but I still went crying to my OB that I could *not* suffer through what I did with number one. Desperation. Serious desperation. I wanted another baby, but I just didn't see how I could manage if I struggled like after my first-born. So that is when I began antidepressants by the name of Zoloft, my friend, or so I thought. Again, this was all normal as far as I understood it all. Many mothers suffer from postpartum depression. It is *normal.* Yet I felt weak, inadequate, and faulty. So this small detail is one that I have mostly kept private, until now.

Then things got scary. Like beyond the *normal* suffering. We got into FUBAR. I was at work at the outpatient orthopedic rehab clinic and was struggling with mild headaches for a few weeks. I had just returned to work two days/week after having my second child in the fall of 2007. I was coasting along with my Zoloft. I remember even a few weeks before that my eyeball hurt. I don't know how to describe it except eyeball pain. I remember being at the local library with my good friend and her two girls during story time. I looked to the extreme and said, "Jen, that was so weird. My eyeball just hurt when I looked to the side. Ha! Motherhood does crazy things to you I guess." She agreed, weird, and then we shrugged it off.

A few weeks passed, and I was at work writing my notes with words like HEP, IADL, etc. I looked up and saw the letters on the building across the parking lot appeared fuzzy. I had begun drinking more coffee in the form of Starbucks Frappuccinos and lattes since I thought caffeine would help me stay awake and decrease the headaches. I had even been treated for a sinus infection near that time. Since moving to the Midwest in 2004, I had started suffering allergies I had never experienced before. I thought it was all the cottonwood that I had never even seen before.

On the way home that day, I had both kids in the car. I had already called my dad about the change in my eyesight. He had said that when vision changes dramatically, I should go see my doctor. This was just one of the many times in the past twelve years I have called my dad for medical advice. On the way home, I covered one of my eyes. I saw the oncoming car disappear and then reappear. Holy crap! What just happened?

Apparently, the insertion of the optic nerve into the optic disc of the retina creates a blind point or scotoma. Although this is considered normal, our brains fill in the missing information, and the spot is not usually noticeable. In optic neuritis (inflammation of the optic nerve), you will have a larger than normal blind spot. Needless to say, off to the emergency room I went.

I saw many doctors. I was admitted to the hospital. I had brain images in the form of MRI, CT, and X-ray. All seemed normal except for this slight swelling in my optic nerve. They ran blood tests; they said words like *multiple sclerosis* and *stroke*. I ended up with a spinal tap to test the pressure of my spinal fluid and its contents. My pressure was slightly elevated, and my white blood count was up, indicating I had increased swelling around my central nervous system and I was fighting an infection. The neuro-ophthalmologist finally diagnosed me with optic neuritis from viral meningitis. Good news is that with rest—and I mean lots of rest—I would recover. Thank goodness! I recovered fully back to my same *normal* as before—fatigue, depression, sinus infections, you know, "normal."

I want to be very clear at this point that at no time did anyone *ever* ask me about my nutritional status. Maybe I tricked them because I *looked* healthy or I *looked* normal. I can tell you for darn sure that optic neuritis and losing vision is *not* normal. I recovered and restored my vision, but nothing about that should ever be considered normal. (See "Epigenetics" for more information about what is considered normal health)

We finished up orthopedic residency and moved back to the Bay Area for my husband's fellowship training. That was a stressful year. We had to endure my husband's ear surgery, removing a cholesteatoma. (This is a skin cell tumor inside the ear canal. It is benign but terribly destructive. No wonder he never heard any of the kids crying at night. "Likely excuse" is what I said.) He had to have two surgeries, one to remove the tumor and the other to put in prosthetic titanium ear bones (malleus, incus, and stapes) so he could hear again. Finally, he landed a *real* job. This was the light at the end of the long tunnel of orthopedic surgery training. Well, let's just say the light looks different than I expected, but we were done. Back to his hometown of Reno, Nevada, we went.

Then the eye pain happened again after my third baby in 2010. I freaked out. I went straight to the neuro-ophthalmologist in town as soon as possible. It took two months, because that is a very specialized field, and apparently there aren't very many. By then, everything was fine again despite my overanalyzing that back in the Midwest they had been wrong about the MS thing. Well, the letters *MS* were thrown around again, but they never did find any plaques on my brain with MRI, nor did my blood work ever show up anything to confirm that diagnosis. It just didn't stick, yet there was no explanation.

During the next few years, Zoloft and I kept things afloat. My toenail fungus was back, but whatever; lots of people had it. But the darn allergies were getting the best of me. In the fall of 2011, I called my father—again. I was struggling with getting good sleep with all the congestion. I had tried over the counter allergy medications, nasal spray, neti pot rinses, peppermint in the shower (I don't recommend breaking a bottle of peppermint in the shower; your eyes and nose will burn like crazy), and even allergy sublingual drops instead of the shots. It seemed *nothing* changed until that phone call to my father. On the phone, as I asked what my next step should be, he said in so many words, "You are morbidly obese and overweight. You need to lose weight, and maybe that will help your sinus problem."

Really? I have given birth to three kids. I don't look like I did when I was living at home. Yes, I was forty-five pounds overweight, but who wasn't? That was *normal*. How could he be so insensitive and hurtful? What I realized in time was that he was trying as best he could. I had called for his opinion, and he had given it to me. It wasn't what I wanted to hear, but he wasn't wrong either. I wasn't morbidly obese. My BMI theoretically was still in the "healthy" range. But if we are totally honest, I wasn't healthy, and I was struggling. What he meant to say, if he had done all the reading that I have now done, was "You are inflamed, and you need to get the inflammation under control."

I completed my McKenzie training in mechanical diagnosis and treatment in 2012. (That is the "Cert MDT" behind my name.) The introduction quote about end-range is specific to getting the painful/deranged joint to end range to get a full reduction or expose any underlying dysfunction. More to the point, it gives you information and a potential for recovery. For me, my father's comments were my "end range." It started me on my journey to discover my own health, because I was no longer satisfied with my "normal."

I had heard of this "paleo diet" before, but I had never dieted before. I loved to eat. As I committed to getting healthy, I started exercising twice a week with a trainer. I needed accountability. I read a book by Robb Wolf, *The Paleo Solution*. Then I read Loren Cordain's books. I started researching on PubMed to be sure this "diet" was, in fact, healthy. I am, of course, a traditionally trained health care provider and need evidence, proof of safety. So many physicians with whom my husband works said, "You are going to get heart disease, eating meat," or "If you take out milk, where are you going to get calcium?" or "If you take away grains, what will you eat?"

In February 2012, I threw away or donated all our bread, all our cereal, all of our nonfat milk, and anything that contained gluten, dairy, sugar or legumes. The data that was presented in the books I read indicated these things were inflammatory. And if it was good for me, it was good for the kids and husband too. God bless my husband for his support because he grew up on pasta and cereal. Not kidding. He didn't even have a salad until his senior year in high school. He wasn't overweight, but healthy isn't quite the word for him given his GERD, chronic upper respiratory infections, and other odd things like ear tumors.

Funny things started to happen as we moved into our paleo-inspired way of life. My allergies dramatically improved. I lost forty-five pounds in six months. My mood improved such that I stopped my antidepressants. (I do not recommend removing antidepressants unless you are under supervision of a doctor.) I began to feel alive. My aches and pains resolved. I had more energy to read, exercise, enjoy life, and simply be connected. It was working for me.

Although this book isn't about my husband's journey specifically (that is for him to share), we did go on this journey together, despite his initial reluctance. I noticed he stopped complaining about hip pain. His mood regulated, and he was less short-tempered with the kids. He stopped taking his Nexium (his medication for heartburn) daily, and it went to only two to three times a year.

Even the kids each had improvements in their health too, fewer upper respiratory infections, and when they did get them, they would recover instead of linger for weeks. Skin conditions improved. Behavior improved. Even my middle child, who had been lactose intolerant with weird aches and pains and even vomiting at times, resolved. They each had a different time frame of change, and each have different symptoms, but all improved. What I had considered normal childhood stuff went away.

For me, it started simply with moving more and then eating well. I then focused on improving my sleep and then moved into purpose and connection, which is what I call *soar*.

All the research articles I found or books I read couldn't have convinced me as much as four direct case studies outside of my immediate nuclear family. The first came when I was working at the local hospital-based outpatient setting. I was working with a fifty-year-old woman who was a librarian at a local school. She was referred to physical therapy to address shoulder stiffness following multiple surgeries related to breast cancer and subsequent infections. During her hospital admission that nearly killed her, she had to be intubated. At that time she was fed through NGT (nasogastric tube) tubes to keep her alive while she was sedated. She was a celiac disease patient, meaning she was allergic to gluten, a specific protein found in wheat products. There is something called cross-reactivity, where proteins in other foods look like the gluten protein and can stimulate the same immune response. Dairy is one of those foods that happen to have proteins that look like gluten called casein. All those feedings she had in the hospital included dairy, and sometimes gluten, which continued to make her sick. Once she was discharged, she was alive with scar tissue limiting her shoulder mobility, and she suffered double vision.

As we worked, I showed her stretches that she had to continue to do to remodel the scar tissue that, over time, would get better. As for the double vision, I couldn't change it, but I could help her body learn to adapt to it to remain balanced. Now that she was out of the hospital, she was cooking for herself and her daughter, being 100% gluten- and dairy-free. After my own personal experience at that time, I just supported and confirmed for her to keep that up, because it mattered. Anything to keep inflammation down would help her recovery, and who knew where she would end up?

A few months passed after she was discharged to her HEP. She called into the clinic to let us know that she had a "miracle" occur. One day she went to the movies with her daughter, and as the movie started, it was like the "curtains went up" and her vision became normal. How cool is that! The way that "miracle" happened was through her consistency with eating whole foods and simply time. Her body finally was able to heal itself. It gives me chills just retelling her story.

The second case was my father-in-law. He suffers from Parkinson's disease, along with many orthopedic and arthritic conditions. Supposedly the Parkinson's is from his exposure to Agent Orange in the Vietnam War, and the arthritic conditions are just genetics. We will never know for sure the absolute cause. He had been home by himself for one week while his wife was on a vacation for three weeks. He was starting to decline, unbeknownst to us, but fortunately, he was able to call my cell phone for help.

He was struggling with his words. When I visited him at his home, it looked like he hadn't taken his medication, nor had he eaten in days. I brought him home to our house and fed him dinner. He came alive again. I set up a food delivery service for the remainder of his wife's trip and got home health services. We modified his medications so they were more manageable, for whatever that was worth. After only a few days of eating paleo-inspired (specifically gluten-free whole foods), he was doing the best we had seen him in years. I work with patients with Parkinson's disease and other autoimmune diseases, and I have never before seen such an improvement, no matter how much we have exercised.

Fortunately, my husband and I went to visit him, and they bantered back and forth about Nevada trivia like they used to. It was beautiful. I specifically remember the smile on not only my father-in-law's face, but also my husband's too. I told my husband that I was happy he had the opportunity to see how good his dad was, because I was sure that the changes we made to his nutrition and activity would not be carried through.

We are all creatures of habit, and as time went on and his wife returned, they both went back to their "normal" nutritional and lifestyle habits. The gains we'd made were only temporary and only sustainable if he continued with the whole foods eating and exercise. It makes me sad every day to know that even with giving them a foundation with the meal delivery and home health to assist with regular exercise, without the reinforcement from all his medical doctors, there was no support in continuing. Not to mention that it is multifactorial, as the four KISS principles will outline. It may start with food, but it isn't the only thing involved.

The fourth encounter was my coworker, Wendy. I will never forget when Wendy called me one evening. Her young daughter had been fighting a lifelong battle with lung infections. Her young daughter had been on and off of medications and breathing treatments for many years of her young life. Her daughter was sick again, and the doctor wanted to do another round of steroids, again. When she called, she asked, "Do you think going paleo would help her?" I encouraged her to try, for she truly had nothing to lose. The worst-case scenario was that nothing would change. The thing is, it actually did. Her daughter's lungs started clearing. The longer they continued whole foods eating, the better she got. The rest of her family noticed improvements too. At the time of writing this book, they recently went hiking at eleven thousand feet. The only complaint their daughter had was that her ankles were sore after climbing the uneven surface for a few miles.

I was so inspired by these few case encounters that I went back to school for a masters of science in holistic nutrition in order to incorporate more detailed lifestyle habits into my physical therapy practice. As part of this journey, I had to complete a case series on a group of people eating whole foods (not pure paleo nor fully organic and non-GMO, but whole foods) for two weeks. I added in a symptom questionnaire and functional questionnaire for those experiencing physical conditions like hip pain or foot pain. The results didn't surprise me, except to further fuel my fire. Every single person experienced improvement in symptoms and pain (except one who actually ate worse during the trial due to travel). The average was a 52.9% improvement in symptoms. That means that by the end of two weeks eating whole foods (as close to nature as possible) they had decreased symptoms, whatever their personal symptoms were, by over 50%. Additionally, those that had a painful condition also had improved their symptoms as they related to quality of life on average by 18%.

It is all about measurable changes and documenting something objective. How much more do I need to see or hear or research before I feel like it is safe? These case studies were new to me, but they are not new for many. If you research many holistic health providers in the paleo community, functional medicine community, and whole foods communities like Weston A Price, you will see similar results.

From where I stand as a health care provider, mother, and wife, the few things I have learned need to be shared. The consequences of ignorance in an easy life and falling prey to marketing are too scary for me. I have worked hard to gain the many tools to help every single patient. Yet I often failed despite my efforts. So I write, I share, and I educate. If writing a book helps just one person to spark his or her own healing or, better yet, prevent disease, then it is all worth it. I hope one day my children will read this book to better understand the choices their father and I made to keep them healthy, and I hope it helps them too.

The purpose of this book is to help people live life. It is not about perfection. Perfection is impossible and an illusion. My father and husband used to say in the operating room, "The enemy of good is better." Striving for perfection often destroys the good work that has already been done and, in the end, is worse than if you had just left it as it was. Obviously, fix it if it is broken, but if things are good, keep them there and be sensitive to changes.

This book is not one big rambling message of all things PubMed and technical speak. There is such a thing as too much information. Not to mention the fact that there is no possible way to know everything about everything from a scientific perspective. So I don't have any randomized, controlled, double-blind study on people living by these four KISS principles. Really, I believe that the best study is a sample size of n = 1, yourself. Bits and pieces have been studied individually. If you want more of the science, feel free to search PubMed or even view my blog to get more science. There is so much out there that it's overwhelming. Many have written books about individual principles, and many keep researching individual components. I would like them to keep doing valuable research. For this book, I would like to synthesize the information in a useable and memorable format so that you, a consumer, a mother, a patient, a health care provider, can fall back on the principles to make a decision in your life on a daily if not hourly basis. The science continues to take care of itself and support all of these KISS principles.

I also believe that the face of change for our country and our world is in the hands of the consumer and parents raising young kids. Once you have an illness and you have developed bad habits, it is much harder to change. It is not impossible, and by all means, I believe every person should *try*. But, once you have an illness or disease, you can make dramatic improvement, but you may never have full recovery. Because the truth is that some changes are permanent. You won't know what those are unless you try to improve by using these principles.

If we can teach all of our children how to live by these KISS principles, we may save them from the devastation of chronic disease and illness. That is worth it.

Keep it simple, stupid, is my mantra, and it does take effort, but it is simple. Change is slow, but it doesn't have to be. Every day we make choices. Having a positive mind-set and a set of positive habits or KISS principles will make it a bit easier. Choosing to take care of yourself and being open-minded to learning will be the face of change for you, your family, our society, and our world.

Triple R Strategy

As I have embarked on this journey of health and sharing, I have tried to incorporate ways to simplify the information. As I was working on writing a section of a chapter for a physical therapy rehabilitation book and heard Jack Johnson's song "Reduce, Reuse, Recycle" from the sound track from a Curious George movie, I thought of "Remove, Replace, Restore." Triple R is an acronym for "Remove, Replace, Restore." It is a strategy to break down a concept into a manageable if not memorable format for education purposes. I use it at the end of every blog I write. I use it with patients. I will use it at the end of every principle I cover.

What Are the Four Principles?

I may have given this away already in the subtitle of the book, but the four KISS principles are as follows:

- Eat well.
- Move well.
- Sleep well.
- Soar on.

The following chapters will discuss each component in more detail and how to bring it all together for a healthy and sustainable lifestyle.

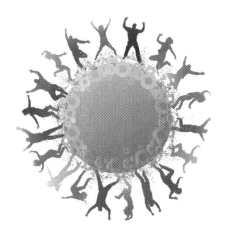

CHAPTER 2: EAT WELL

Cooking (from scratch) is the single most important thing we could do as a family to improve our health and general well being.

—Michael Pollan

What Is Real Food?

To put it simply, to *eat well*, you must eat *real food*, not something that only looks like food. Most of the food you eat must be in its natural or whole form, free of contamination, in order to maximize nutrient-richness and absorption. However, in today's world, understanding what real food is has become a bit confusing.

Real food is as close to its natural state as possible. It is *simple*. It is in its whole form and merely needs to be eaten or cooked for consumption and for the nutrients to be absorbed by the body. An example of real food would be broccoli. Broccoli can be safely eaten raw, or it can be gently cooked. An apple can also be eaten raw or cooked. The bioavailability of nutrients in a whole food is optimal for natural absorption.

In case there is any confusion about what exactly is a whole food, below is a chart listed in order of decreasing nutrient-richness adapted from George Mateljan's *The World's Healthiest Foods*: [2]

VEGETABLES		POULTRY AND	Corn
Spinach	Cantaloupe	LEAN MEATS	
Swiss Chard	Pineapple	Calf's Liver	HERBS AND
Mushrooms	Kiwi Fruit	Beef, Grass-fed	SPICES
Asparagus	Oranges	Venison	Parsley
Brocoli	Papaya	Lamb	Mustard Seeds
Romaine Lettuce	Watermelon	Chicken	Basil
Collard Greens	Apricots	Turkey	Turmeric
Kale/Mustard	Grapefruit		Cinnamon
Greens	Grapes	BEANS AND	Cayenne Pepper
Tomatoes	Blueberries	LEGUMES**	Black Pepper
Brussel Sprouts	Cranberries	Lentils	Ginger
Green Beans	Bananas	Soybeans	Dill
Squash	Plum	Kidney Beans	Cilantro
Bell Peppers	Lemons	Lima Beans	Rosemary
Cauliflower	Limes	Black Beans	
Celery/Fennel	Apples	Garbanzo Beans	
Green Peas	Figs	Tofu	FATS
Cabbage	Pears	Dried Peas	For heat:
Carrots		Peanuts	Butter
Winter Squash	FISH AND		Ghee (Clarified
Beets	SHELLFISH *	DAIRY*** AND	butter)
Eggplant	Tuna	EGGS****	Tallow
Garlic	Shrimp	Eggs	Lard
Onions/Leeks	Salmon	Whole Milk	Coconut oil
Sweet Potatoes	Cod	Yogurt (no sugar	
Cucumbers	Sardines	added)	For low heat:
Potatoes	Scallops	Cheese	Cold pressed Olive
Avocados		Goat's Milk	oil
Sea Vegetables	NUTS AND SEEDS		
Shiitake	Sunflower Seeds	GRAINS**	Unheated only:
Mushrooms	Flaxseeds	Oats	Cold pressed seed
Olives	Sesame Seeds	Rye	oils (ie walnut)
	Pumpkin Seeds	Quinoa	
FRUITS	Walnuts	Brown Rice	Fermented cod
Strawberries	Almonds	Whole Wheat	liver oil
Raspberries	Cashews	Buckwheat	

*Wild Caught Preferred
**Whole organic, non-GMO, traditionally prepared, soaked overnight if consuming
***Organic, whole raw milk if possible if consuming
****Organic, free-range preferred

Table 1: Whole foods listed in order of decreasing nutrient-richness.

It seems easy enough to eat real food and eat just enough for your active lifestyle, not too much and not too little. Eat when you are hungry and stop when you are full.

Remove. Replace. Restore.
Remove food-like substances.
Replace with *real* food.
Restore health.

Water

We forget that the water cycle and the life cycle are one.

—Jacques Cousteau

Water is life. Yet it is often forgotten. Water is an important macronutrient that acts as a biological solvent, transport medium, or lubricant for other nutrients. Water provides a chemical reactant for biochemical reactions like hydrolysis (chemical bonds broken) and condensation (producing water). Water also facilitates regulation of body temperature. The process for regulation, fluid balance, is by means of electrolytes like NaCl (salt) that occur through the process of osmosis (movement across cell membranes, either passively or selectively). [3] This process is also carefully regulated by way of blood volume by the brain and kidneys via the aldosterone produced by the adrenal glands and the antidiuretic hormone produced in the pituitary gland. Water is critical for the absorption of the nutrients in your whole foods as well as for keeping your physiological processes going.

The bigger question is, "How much water do you need to drink?" Like most questions, there isn't a black and white answer, only a concept of simplicity. There are two extremes here. Both are extremely rare but worth understanding.

Dehydration is also called hypohydration and is a disruption of the metabolic process as a result of the body not having enough water. This occurs when the water loss is greater than water intake as can occur with excessive exercise, in certain climates, and from failing to consume enough fluids in the forms of pure water and metabolic water in fruits and vegetables. Symptoms of dehydration with a 3–4% decrease in body water are fatigue and dizziness. An over 10% decrease in body water causes symptoms to progress into mental and physical deterioration as well as severe thirst. An above 15% decrease in body water is often fatal. These cases require medical attention. The symptoms of the mild form of dehydration, which is common, primarily include thirst. Drinking oral fluids is sufficient to rehydrate water volume.

Hyponatremia, or overhydration, is a condition of low blood sodium as a result of excessive water consumption. This too is often fatal. A case study was published about the death of a female hiker in the Grand Canyon as a result of hyponatremia. [4] This woman had completed a five-hour hike into the canyon and shortly collapsed and died afterward. Her attempts to stay hydrated in such a severe condition resulted in overhydration, and losing her water-electrolyte balance resulted in her death. Again, this is an extreme case, but there are many reports of fatalities with overhydration in athletes.[5]

The Institute of Medicine has outlined adequate intakes for total water intake. [6] Below is a chart summary of their recommendations:

Age	Total water intake (L)	Fluid (beverage intake) (L)
0–6 mos.	0.7	0.7
7–12 mos.	0.8	0.8
1–3 years	1.3	0.9
4–8 years	1.7	1.2
9–11 years		
Boys	2.4	1.8
Girls	2.1	1.6
>14 years as adults		
Boys	3.3	2.6
Girls	2.3	1.8
Adults		
Men	3.3	2.6
Women	2.3	1.8
Pregnant women	+0.3	0.1
Lactating women	+1.10	0.90
Elderly	As adults	As adults

Table 2: Water intake recommendations from
the Institute of Medicine (IOM)

It is sometimes recommended by health advocates to "drink half your body weight in ounces of water daily." Although this recommendation is a little higher than the IOM recommendations, it is not validated by research per se. I have also heard, "Drink enough water until your urine runs clear," or "Don't wait until you are thirsty to drink." These recommendations have been linked to overhydration in marathon athletes and potentially risk hyponatremia or death.[5]

Although I present a few extreme cases here, the bigger issue is that all of those statements take the individual out of the equation. Teaching someone to listen to his or her body is the safest and best way to achieve water balance. You can definitely have too much of a good thing and not enough of a vital component.

Balance is critical. Anything can become destructive if you don't pay attention to balance. Not too little. Not too much. If we *listen* to our bodies, we can achieve *balance*. Drink fresh water when you are thirsty and stop when you are satiated.

Remove. Replace. Restore.

Remove being ignorant about your own body's signals.

Replace with moderation. Not too little. Not too much. Listen to your body. Drink when you are thirsty. Stop when you are satiated. Exercise regularly but avoid extreme conditions.

Restore water balance.

Refined and Processed

The whole is more than the sum of its parts.

—Aristotle

Packaged foods are often refined and processed. A refined food is a reduced version of the original whole food. It has been mechanically or chemically processed, resulting in the removal of many of the food's original nutrients. The more refined the food, the fewer nutrients remain. In many cases, this is even considered negative nutrition. That means the substance provides no nutrients *to* the body but requires stored nutrients *from* the body to process. Many refined and processed foods can have additives, preservatives, or flavor enhancers. Because of this, it is important to read labels on *everything* in a package.

Some processed foods can be very nutritious. For example, fresh juicing removes the fiber and pulp from the fruits and vegetables but leaves a vitamin- and mineral-rich juice that is easily and rapidly absorbed. It even matters how oil is processed. In order to maintain the integrity and nutrients of oils, it must be expeller-expressed and unrefined in order to preserve the integrity of the fatty acids. Grains and legumes are *inedible* unless they are soaked, fermented, and sprouted to reduce phytic acid (a process that is often skipped altogether in mass production of refined grains in the form of flour). There will be more on fats, grains, and legumes later in the "Inflammation" section.

Here is a list of foods to be cautious of. I consider many of these types of foods to be negative-nutrition foods, meaning that not only are they processed and refined in a manner that removes potential nutrients, but also that they require your body's stored nutrients to process and you get none in return. Additionally, the refining process can even make the food look like a "foreign substance" to the body. When your body encounters something foreign, it stimulates an immune response, which complicates things even further. For example, when dairy is pasteurized, it destroys the natural enzymes that actually assist in digestion and absorption. When fat is removed, it leaves a white liquid that is primarily sugar, also known as lactose. Although this process of pasteurization prevents bacteria transmission, it leaves a product devoid of nutrients and requires nutrients from the body to process. It doesn't even look like milk to the body anymore. Yet fermenting dairy in the form of yogurt, kefir, or cheese helps break down the proteins and sugars so the dairy is more readily digested. There will be more on dairy in the "Inflammation" section.

Negative Nutrition Foods (aka Not Real Food)

- Crackers
- Cookies
- Chips
- Tortillas
- Pasteurized or boxed juice (fresh-squeezed juice is nutrient-rich)
- Bread
- Nonfat/low-fat milk
- Donuts
- Protein powders
- Soda (regular or diet)
- Sugar
- Artificial sweetener (NutraSweet)
- High-fructose corn syrup
- Trans-fatty acids (canola oil, hydrogenated vegetable oil, crackers, pastries, shortening, margarine—be aware when eating out)

In the end, the safest choice is always to choose something that is minimally processed or refined. If it does need to be refined or processed, just be aware of how it is done so you know whether that item is retaining its nutrients or not. When a process actually improves nutrients, like fermentation, then enjoy. Eat negative-nutrition foods sparingly. Our vitamin/mineral balance is fragile at best. Make it a habit to eat nutrient-rich whole foods, and you will be doing your body good and helping with disease prevention.

Remove. Replace. Restore.
Remove negative-nutrition foods.
Replace with *whole* nutrient-rich foods.
Restore health.

Why Does Organic, Non-GMO, Grass-Fed Matter?

Quality means doing it right when no one is looking.

—Henry Ford

While weight loss is important, what's more important is the quality of food you put in your body—food is information that quickly changes your metabolism and genes.

—Mark Hyman, MD

One of my husband's physiology professors in medical school said that instead of saying, "I love you with all my heart," we should say, "I love you with all my *liver*." He didn't mean that the heart wasn't an amazing organ, except to say that the liver may be even more amazing. For me, I often say that no system or organ operates in isolation. What is bad for one system likely has detrimental effects on another. We just haven't researched yet to identify. For example, we have all heard of fatty liver disease in alcoholics. Does that mean that there isn't any neurological or cardiovascular effect? No, of course not. It affects the whole body and all systems.

The liver has many vital functions. To name just a few vital functions, the liver stores vitamins and nutrients like glycogen and fat, produces bile that helps digest fat, regulates metabolism, produces proteins to help in clotting, and even regenerates itself after injury.[7] The role of the liver, the great detoxifier, is critical to life, and it is this role I think the professor was referring to. Detoxification, the removal of waste material, is essential to the healthy function of all of our body systems. The liver is our great detoxifier that filters *all* substances that are absorbed through the digestive system into the bloodstream.

Organic means that synthetic pesticides and chemical fertilizers are not allowed in the production chain, nor is irradiation, nor industrial solvents. The United States Department of Agriculture (USDA) regulates the labeling of organic products. So if you are eating nonorganic foods, that means there is likely other pesticides and chemicals potentially on or in the food that your liver has to work extra hard to filter out. Now, organic foods are likely more expensive, and if you need to limit spending due to finances, then the Environmental Working Group (EWG) has developed the "Dirty Dozen" (a list of the fruits and vegetables that contain the highest amounts of pesticides and that should always be bought organic). Additionally, EWG also developed the "Clean Fifteen" (a list of fruits and vegetables that contain the least amount of pesticides).

Dirty Dozen	Clean Fifteen
Apples	Asparagus
Celery	Avocados
Cherry tomatoes	Cabbage
Cucumbers	Cantaloupe
Grapes	Cauliflower
Nectarines	Eggplant
Peaches	Grapefruit
Potatoes	Kiwi
Snap Peas	Mangoes
Spinach/kale/collard greens	Onions
Strawberries	Papayas
Sweet bell peppers/hot peppers	Pineapples
	Sweet corn
	Sweet potatoes
	Sweet peas

Table 3: The "Dirty Dozen" (highest pesticide residue, buy organic) and "Clean Fifteen" (least pesticide residue, safe nonorganic) fruits and vegetables, courtesy of www.ewg.org.

Grass-fed and organic meats also can decrease the burden on your liver, not to mention that they are better for the environment. Grass-fed animals gain valuable nutrients by eating what they are designed to eat versus things like corn, which is not natural to their diet nor digestion and ends up draining nutrients from the animal in order to process. This results in fewer nutrients for you when you consume that animal. There is additional burden on your body, should the animal be exposed to pesticides.

A genetically modified organism (GMO) is an organism that has altered genetic material. The history of genetic modification began with selective breeding. Think of the Labradoodle, the breeding of a Labrador retriever with a standard poodle. They are crossed to produce a medium-sized dog with fur that is allergen-free. As it relates to food, this crossbreeding can even occur from one flowering plant to another by pure chance from an encounter with a bee. Another way is to selectively cross two types of apple trees to produce one that has robust roots to sustain harsher winters. In today's food system, it starts to get more complicated as we go from natural selection to selective crossbreeding to bioengineering. Bioengineering to genetically modify organisms often is used to produce maximum growth and to prevent microbes or insects from affecting the plant during growth. In some cases, the GMO food involves not only selective breeding but also modifying the DNA to incorporate viruses or even pesticides into the genetic material of the food. I understand the need for them as far as farming goes in order to mass-produce food, as I have struggled to grow a tomato in my home garden. However, in introducing the GMO food into our human food chain, it seems obvious to me that what may kill insects or bugs, would likely have some effect on the human body, which is also a living organism. There is no safe level of consumption recommendation of this per se, but it may be impossible to avoid altogether. Either way, it is still better to eat an apple over the highly refined and processed candy bar, GMO or not.

Remove. Replace. Restore.
Remove non-organic and GMO food.
Replace with organic, grass-fed, non-GMO whole foods.
Restore health.

Inflammation

> Researchers have known for some time now that the cornerstone of all degenerative conditions, including brain disorders, is inflammation.

—David Perlmutter, MD, *Grain Brain*

Inflammation is the body's response to an injury or infection. This can be localized or systemic. When the inflammatory response is systemic, it can be potentially life threatening. (For example, think: anaphylactic shock from a bee sting for someone allergic to bees.) Most inflammatory responses, both systemic and localized, are not deadly. They often even run undetected or at a low grade to merely disrupt the normal balance. (Think: mosquito bite or even a mild sprained ankle.) The severity of the inflammation response merely indicates the necessity of either *immediate* medical attention (anaphylactic shock) or support to healing, recovery, and prevention of reinjury/reexposure.

As this relates to food, I want to review a few food items that have been linked to systemic inflammatory responses. There have been higher rates of allergy (strong inflammatory responses that often leads to anaphylaxis requiring immediate medical intervention) for milk, eggs, peanuts, tree nuts, fish, shellfish, soy, and wheat. [8] Lectins in legumes like soy and peanuts are what are primarily responsible for most allergic reactions. [7] In 2007, three million children are reported to have food allergies, and 90% of the allergies are due to the foods listed above.

If you look at most of the list, many of those food items are heavily processed, refined, or mass-produced. For example, most standard dairy is heavily processed, refined, and heated, and the fat has been removed, resulting in a sugary white fluid that looks nothing like it should naturally. That also includes removing enzymes and bacteria present in raw milk that assist in digestion. Your body does not know how to process this sugary white fluid and likely produces a subclinical (you don't notice) inflammatory response initially. Over time, more obvious symptoms may arise with continued exposure.

Let's look at wheat in the form of flour, a staple that makes up a substantial majority of the standard American diet (used for cereal, bread, pasta, etc.). A specific protein called gluten in wheat, barley, rye, and possibly oats has been strongly linked to an allergic reaction in many adults called celiac disease. [3] The gluten protein damages the absorptive surface of the small intestine, making it difficult to absorb nutrients from food. Luckily for those with gluten allergy, there is a test that makes celiac disease relatively simple to diagnose and manage, yet it is still disruptive to your lifestyle.

What if your inflammatory response isn't in the allergic range? What happens then? A nonimmunological reaction to a substance in food is called food intolerance (or food sensitivity). An example of this would be lactose intolerance. The common reaction to this would be stomach cramps or loose stools when ingesting milk. If we look at the gluten protein again, what happens when you aren't allergic, but your inflammatory response is *not* digestive in nature? It is possible to have a reaction anywhere in the body, like depression, anxiety, sleep disturbance, joint pain, fatigue, and even acne.

Studies done by Dickerson in 2010 showed a link to gluten sensitivity and psychiatric brain disorders like schizophrenia, [9] acute mania, [10] and bipolar disorders[11] without celiac disease (gluten *allergy*). We can speculate about the cause of this, but the point really is this: just because you don't have an allergic reaction or a gastrointestinal problem does *not* mean that you have *no* reaction. The inflammatory reaction could be anywhere in your body. A few studies have linked gluten allergy or sensitivity to diseases like systemic lupus erythematous,[12]connective tissue disease, [13] back pain, [14] rheumatoid arthritis, [15] and ankylosing spondylitis. [16] One author described a case study of a forty-year-old woman with a three-week history of left-knee pain and swelling that responded to a gluten-free diet, stretching, and strengthening, demonstrating the potential role of gluten in joint inflammation. [17] You are lucky if you have a gastrointestinal reaction, because it is more obvious. *Do not* ignore the reaction anywhere else, like depression, anxiety, sleep disturbance, joint pain, fatigue, or even acne, to name a few.

There are a few other common inflammatory components in our processed foods that should be avoided. One is refined sugar and artificial sweeteners; the other is trans-fatty acids. Sugar is a no-brainer, yet it is a challenging one. Sugar ingestion stimulates the pancreas to release the hormone insulin, which also regulates inflammation pathways. So the more sugar you ingest, the higher your insulin level, and therefore, there is an increase in inflammation. Sugar can come in the forms of high-fructose corn syrup, fructose, sucrose, rice syrup, turbinado sugar, raw sugar, agave, maltose, dextrose, and many others. The best way to avoid it is to remove prepackaged foods and drinks from your diet.

High sugar consumption has been linked to rheumatoid arthritis, [18] depression, [19] and metabolic disorders like diabetes, stroke, and obesity, which also have links to osteoarthritis[20] and decreased immune function by slowing neutrophil cell [21] and cartilage degradation. [22] Metabolic disorders are also associated with high inflammatory markers and a decreased rehabilitation potential from stroke. [23] The World Health Organization (WHO) recommends that a normal body-mass index adult take in only 25 g/day, or 6 tsp. [24] The average amount of sugar in some popular yogurt with fruit is about 15 g/serving. The average soda contains 40 g of sugar. An average granola bar has 12 g of sugar. That's 67 g sugar just on snacks. The WHO recommends that the free sugars should be less than 10% of total energy intake and that further reduction to 5% would provide additional health benefits. [24] Sugar clearly makes life more complicated and does not fit within the KISS principle of eat well.

What about artificial sweeteners? Well, they too are not natural and complicate the situation. The effect of artificial sweeteners occurs as inflammation in the gut by disrupting the homeostasis we have with our microbiome. [25] (See "Microbiome and Bugs.")

Another inflammatory food product is trans-fatty acid. Trans-fatty acid is an industrially produced, partially hydrogenated vegetable oil. Examples of trans-fatty acids are canola oil, shortening, vegetable oil or margarine. It is often included in packaged snacks like crackers, chips, and pastries. It is often used for deep frying as well. High consumption of trans-fatty acids has been linked to an inflammatory condition called heart disease. [26] It has been associated with inflammatory conditions of the neurological system[27] and integumentary (skin and hair) system. [28] Nutritional researchers have not identified an allowable or even safe recommended dose of trans-fatty acids for human consumption. [29] Without a doubt, trans-fatty acids make life more complicated and, therefore, do not meet the KISS criteria.

Below, table 4 summarizes some of the dietary contributors to systemic inflammation, the food in which it is found, and the potential system response. Later, we will discuss those nutritional components that reverse inflammation in the "Healing" section.

Dietary limitations/ avoidance	Food in which Found	Inflammatory Response
Carbohydrates[30-34]	Candies, desserts, flour-derived baked or processed foods, pastas, cereals, granola, fruit juice, beans/legumes, dried fruits (especially if sweetened), anything with added sugars	Neurologic, inflammatory microbiota
Fructose[35-37]	Agave syrup, honey, dates, raisins, dried fruit, molasses, green grapes, canned fruit in syrup, fruit juice	Metabolic syndrome, decrease osteogenesis/ skeletal bone growth, increase neutrophils glycation end products
Aspartame[38-45]	NutraSweet, Equal, a potential additive in sweet-tasting, "sugar-free" foods	Carpal tunnel syndrome, disrupts microbiome, rheumatoid arthritis, mitochondrial death, neurological free radical damage, glucose intolerance, memory deficits, liver inflammation
Ethanol[46]	Beer, wine, spirits, mixed adult beverages	IGF-1 growth hormone, fatty liver disease

Monosodium glutamate[47,48]	MSG, may be present in an ingredient list as "flavoring," processed packaged foods, restaurant foods	Neurological, mechanical sensitization
Gliadin (gluten protein)[9,49]	Wheat, oats, barley (anything containing gluten)	Celiac disease, increase IL-15 in noncoeliac
Statins[50]	Consult physician	Tendon weakness
NSAIDs (Nonsteroidal anti-inflammatory like Advil, Motrin)[51]	Consult physician	Tendon weakness
Birth control[52-54]	Consult physician	Disrupts microbiome, IGF-1 growth hormone
Trans fats[26-28,55,56]	Vegetable and seed oils (Canola, rape seed, soybean, safflower, partially hydrogenated fat/oil)	Gastrointestinal inflammation, heart disease, neurological, skin damage, decrease dopamine neurons
Advanced glycation end products[57]	Charred meats, high dietary sugar/carbohydrate intake	Increase tendon stiffness

Table 4: Nutritional components found to exacerbate inflammation and the foods to avoid. Above referenced foods found on government website http://ndb.nal.usda.gov/.

Unnatural, engineered food products produce inflammatory responses in the body across all systems. This, by definition, is not simple, and in fact, we would be ill advised to continue consuming unlimited amounts or even to allow them in our food chain.

You may wonder if remaining gluten-free, limiting dairy and legumes, and eating whole nutrient-dense foods, including healthy fat and protein, is safe. Dr. Terry Wahls, MD, who used nutritional and functional medicine principles to reverse her own multiple sclerosis, has performed and continues to perform clinical studies on patients with progressive multiple sclerosis (MS) for the "Wahls Protocol." This protocol includes a specific eating strategy to avoid inflammatory foods and specific inclusion of anti-inflammatory and nutrient-rich whole foods. In order to carry out clinical studies in humans, you must first demonstrate that your treatment will do no harm. [58] The initial results are promising in reducing levels of fatigue in patients with MS, a hallmark symptom of multiple sclerosis.

Avoiding inflammatory foods is a safe way to eat.

Remove. Replace. Restore.

Remove inflammatory foods: refined sugars; refined grains, especially gluten; artificial sweeteners; and trans-fatty acids like margarine.

Replace with whole organic fruits and vegetables and healthy fats from grass-fed organic meat, butter, olive oil, fish oil.

Restore healthy inflammatory responses and health.

Epigenetics

Genes load the gun, but environment pulls the trigger.

—Bruce Lipton, PhD

You said what? Yes, this is a complicated word with a simple meaning.

Epigenetics is essentially how we turn our genes on without changing the DNA sequence. Our genes can be turned on by environmental factors that include how we move, how we sleep, what we breathe, and yes, what we eat. What you eat directly effects how your genetic makeup is expressed. So illnesses like heart disease, osteoarthritis, autoimmune diseases like Parkinson's, multiple sclerosis, and rheumatoid arthritis all are more likely to be expressed if turned on by a specific environmental factor.

GMO foods, especially those foods that are genetically engineered, put a bit of a complication in the epigenetic expression. There are a lot of social movements and chatter that says genetically modified organisms (with altered DNA, not simply crossbreeding) when ingested disrupt how our genes are turned on. Doesn't that make perfect sense? It does to me. This is why there is so much lobbying around GMO labeling and organic labeling too, appropriately so. In an effort to mass-produce food-like substances, we have sacrificed our own genetic expression.

Yet, if you change the environmental factor, like nutrition, you essentially turn the same gene on but in a better way. So just because your father and grandfather had severe hip osteoarthritis does not mean you are destined for the same fate. By avoiding foods that cause inflammation and that negatively affect your gene expression and by eating natural foods that turn your genes on normally, you may find that your hips don't develop osteoarthritis like your father. You can improve your genetic expression by eating well (and moving well, sleeping well, and soaring). This correction in your gene expression today will be passed on as an improvement in your offspring if done before having children. That is pretty cool.

A series of studies done by Francis M. Pottenger, Jr, MD, in cats, demonstrated the effects of a poor, processed diet on the health of cats and their offspring over several generations. Additionally, the health of Pottenger's cats was restored, including that of their offspring, when diet was restored to a one that was natural to their species and in its purest and most wholesome form. [59] The epigenetic expression of the genes in these cats was directly affected by what the cats ate, and subsequent generations reaped the benefits of good nutrition.

I certainly hope that I caught my kids' epigenetic expression in time for them to turn on their genes in the most optimal way and that my grandchildren will be even better off. Our family genetic code predicts that if they don't, they could have cardiovascular disease, diabetes, Parkinson's disease, dementia, osteoarthritis, glaucoma, and other unknown diseases. Yet changing how they eat at such a young age truly has the epigenetic expression for improved health today and for the future if they choose to keep it up.

Remove. Replace. Restore.
Remove nutrient deficient and inflammatory foods.
Replace with whole, organic, non-GMO produce and meat.
Restore genetic wealth and beauty and health.

Leaky Gut

Anything that affects the gut will always affect the brain.

—Dr. Charles Majors

Digestion begins in the mouth. Food then passes into your esophagus and then into the stomach where it meets with gastric juices to initiate breakdown of food into smaller particles for absorption in the small intestine before exiting through the large intestine out the rectum as stool. Primary nutrient and mineral absorption occurs in the small intestine. This is also the primary barrier to guard your body from invaders. It is also said that 90% of your immunity lies in the small intestine.[7]

Within the small intestine, there are millions of microvilli lining the intestinal wall. This barrier has a paradoxical role in that it allows nutrients to pass into the bloodstream while providing a barrier for foreign substances (like chemicals, bacterial products, and large molecules).[7] When this barrier is disrupted by excessive consumption of processed foods (especially those that include gluten from wheat), sugar, alcohol, medications like nonsteroidal anti-inflammatories (NSAIDS), or lectins (found in legumes), the gut loses its integrity and, therefore, loses its control over what comes in.[7] This inability to absorb nutrients properly is a condition called "leaky gut." The cellular junctions that were once tightly connected now allow food particles into the body. Your body responds by producing an inflammatory response against the foreign particles. Scientific literature and studies continue to verify this phenomenon, especially in those who also have neurological symptoms and autoimmune diseases.[10,11,60,61]

This condition is reversible with time, adequate whole foods nutrition, including healing fats, avoiding the foods and medications that aggravate the condition, and restoring the microbiome with fermented foods or probiotics.[62] (See "Microbiome and Bugs.") I should also emphasize that the ability for your gut junctions to open and close is actually normal. It is abnormal for us to keep them open indefinitely as we often do with traditional medication use and the SAD diet.

Remove. Replace. Restore.

Remove refined sugars, refined grains (especially those containing gluten), refined vegetable oils (trans-fatty acids like margarine), artificial sweeteners, and minimize medications if possible by consulting with a physician.

Replace with whole, organic, non-GMO produce and organic, grass-fed, wild meat, as well as healthy fats and probiotic foods to reinoculate the gut.

Restore gut integrity, your immunity, and your health.

Microbiome and Bugs

All disease begins in the gut.

—Hippocrates

These good guys are little bacteria that live in your gut that we live with harmoniously. Altogether, they number in the millions in your mouth, up to billions in your small intestine, and there are trillions in your large intestine. This army of little ones acts like an organ and, in large part, is the immune system that keeps you from getting sick. This teeny army protects us from unfriendly bacteria and parasites. They even manufacture nutrients for us like vitamin K and B-complex vitamins.[7]

Each of us has a different makeup to our little army that is a result of how we were born (vaginal or C-section), whether or not we were breast-fed, if we played in the dirt when we were kids, what we eat, and even other lifestyle factors. The little bugs feed off the food you ingest. The standard American diet high in simple carbohydrates, and sugar tends to preferentially feed unhealthy yeast and bacteria, not the beneficial fighting bugs.

Another medication that can directly affect our quality of microbiome is antibiotic use. Antibiotics kill bugs. Sometimes we need them to kill scary bugs to stay alive. Once our life is saved, then it is time to get our good bugs back, which may mean eating more fermented probiotic foods like sauerkraut, kimchi, kombucha, pickles, yogurt, or a professional-grade probiotic supplement. Healthy doses of fiber in the form of vegetables and fruit also help support the little guys. Professional-grade probiotic supplements tend to be more reliable as they come refrigerated to keep the bugs alive. Additionally, the professional grade probiotics will often have a higher concentration in the billions that is required to reinoculate the intestinal system after disruption or illness.

Some of the friendliest bacteria that have been identified that even help with disease prevention are: [63]

- *Lactobacillis plantarum*;
- *Lactobacillus acidophilus*;
- *Bifidobacterium breve*; and
- *Bifidobacterium longum*.

More friendly bacteria continue to be discovered today.

What disrupts the bug's balance? It happens to be many of the same things that cause inflammation. Disrupters of the balance are refined sugar, refined grains, medications (especially antibiotics and birth control), [64] artificial sweeteners, trans-fatty acids, chlorine, and, of course, pesticides. All of these little army fighters help keep us healthy, and the best food for them is whole organic produce, organic meats, and wild-caught seafood.

Restoring your fighting gut bugs is associated with healing illness, including leaky gut, and restoring balance. Please restore your fighting bugs and feed them plenty of fiber from whole produce.

Remove. Replace. Restore.

Remove refined sugar, artificial sweetener, refined grains, trans-fatty acids, chlorinated water, and medications (when safe and with a doctor's supervision).

Replace with whole organic produce, grass-fed/wild meat and fish, filtered water, probiotic-rich fermented foods like sauerkraut, kimchi, pickles, and yogurt, and probiotic supplementation if needed.

Restore the army of bugs that protect you from invaders and provide you with valuable nutrients.

Fat (Not Make You Fat)

We cannot solve our problems with the same thinking we used when we created them.

—Albert Einstein

Fats are also called lipids. Fats are an important macronutrient that supplies concentrated energy for your body, support cellular health, and aid vitamin and mineral absorptions. Unlike the old adage that fats are bad for you and that animal fats lead to heart attack, healthy consumption is actually health-promoting and brain-supporting. In order to absorb fat-soluble vitamins, you need fat. Fat-soluble vitamins include vitamins A, D, E, and K. Many of these fat-soluble vitamins, especially vitamins A, D, and K2, work synergistically together to maintain bone health[65] but are even found in animal fats that we tend to avoid. Not only that, but lipids are the precursor to many hormones that support our metabolic processes.

The human fat cell also has another cool feature called transdifferentiation. This process describes the ability of a fat cell to turn into a muscle cell or a bone cell and then back again. Depending on the signals you send, an adipocyte (human fat cell) can then be turned into something else, as it is needed, be it muscle, bone, nerve, skin cell, or stem cell. The fat cell has plasticity, the ability to change. [66-68] If you want to make your muscles bigger, your bones stronger, and even your brain smarter, you want fat present in your diet so you can then make it work to your benefit, especially when healing from an injury or recovering from illness.

What makes a fat good or bad? To answer this question we need to look at the fundamentals. Lipids that are called oils are liquid at room temperature, while those that are solid at room temperature are called fats. Lipids come in the form of fatty acids, triglycerides, phospholipids, and sterols. They are named based on the number of carbon atoms and the number and position of double bonds. Saturated fatty acid (SFA) has all single carbon–carbon bonds, and unsaturated fatty acids (UFA) contain one or more double bonds. The position of the hydrogen bond determines whether it is bent (cis-fatty acid) or straight (trans-fatty acid).

Saturated fatty acids (SFA) are primarily from animal sources and are considered stable and solid at room temperature. The stability indicates that their shape doesn't change when they are heated.

Sources of high SFA

- Mother's breast milk
- Coconut oil
- Lard (beef fat, pork fat)
- Butter
- Palm oil

Unsaturated fatty acids (UFA) can be monounsaturated or polyunsaturated. The more double bonds present, the more bends that occur, indicating the potential to change. Unsaturated fatty acids tend to be liquid at room temperature and are considered oils. They tend to be more fragile and heat sensitive.

Sources of high unsaturated fatty acids (UFA)

- Canola oil
- Safflower oil
- Sunflower oil
- Corn oil
- *Olive oil**
- Soybean oil
- Margarine
- *Fish oil**

*See below for associated positive health benefits.

Unsaturated fatty acids can be further categorized into trans or cis, depending on the location of the hydrogen atoms around the double bond. The cis form has two hydrogen atoms on the same side of the double bond, which results in a bend, whereas the trans form has the hydrogen atoms on opposite sides, resulting in a straight fatty acid. Therefore, the trans-fatty acids (TFA) are more likely to be solid at room temperature. This occurs *naturally* in some fats like dairy and beef. However, this most *commonly* occurs commercially via the process of partial hydrogenation. You see this in margarine and shortening used for baking. It produces a desirable texture and reduces spoiling. The main sources of TFA in our diet are in baked items and for deep-frying.

Sources of high trans-fatty acids (TFA)

- Canola oil
- Hydrogenated vegetable oil
- Partially hydrogenated vegetable oil
- Crackers (often hidden ingredient for texture)
- Pastries
- Shortening
- Margarine (soft butter spreads)

Why does this matter? Incorporating lipids (fat) is essential for cellular health, cellular energy, vitamin absorption, and hormone production. However, industrialized high TFA is actually detrimental to health. There has been a causal link associated with TFA consumption from partially hydrogenated vegetable oil and cardiovascular disease. A systematic review and meta-analysis study distinguished between ruminant TFA (that which occurs naturally in beef or dairy) and industrial TFA (partially hydrogenated vegetable oils, for example). The conclusions support that industrial TFA is positively related to heart disease, while ruminant TFA was not. [26]

Another review article supported these findings but noted that there was no lower limit that has been found to be safe as far as ingestion of industrialized TFA. In fact, consumption of the TFA that occurs naturally in beef and dairy seems to have minimal cardiovascular risk when consumed with a balanced diet. [29]

I often emphasize the fact that our body systems never act in isolation and, in fact, work in a complementary way. It is no surprise that recovering from a sports injury still requires remodeling of neural pathways related to motor learning. In relation to TFA, there have been studies that indicate that consumption of industrialized TFA can negatively affect other body systems, including the neurological and integumentary system.

The *neurological system* is negatively affected by industrialized TFA. In fact an animal study done by Trevizol et al. in 2015, demonstrated a link between consumption of hydrogenated vegetable fat (high in industrialized TFA) and neurological changes that corresponded to hyperactive behavior, oxidative damage, and molecular changes that may lead to development of neuropsychiatric conditions like bipolar disorder. [27]

Even the *integumentary system,* which includes skin and hair, is negatively impacted by industrialized TFA consumption. Barcelos et al. in 2014 performed an animal study to measure the effects of soybean oil, fish oil, and hydrogenated vegetable fat (high-industrialized TFA). They fed pregnant rats the different oils and maintained them through breast-feeding. They then observed the skin of the offspring as it responded to ultraviolet exposure. They found that fish oil was protective of the offspring's skin to ultraviolet radiation exposure. However, the group receiving industrialized TFA offspring showed increased skin wrinkles, reactive oxygen species, and decreased mitochondrial integrity and glutathione levels, the master antioxidant of the body. Altogether, that makes the skin prone to develop photoaging and skin cancer. [28]

As Barcelos showed, consumption of fish oil (a naturally occurring fatty acid) demonstrated protective qualities to the skin from skin cancer, other studies have also shown positive effects of fish oil and olive oil (naturally occurring unsaturated fatty acids). Marques demonstrated that supplementation with fish oil reduces markers of muscle damage, inflammatory disturbances, and neutrophil death that is induced by intensive exercise. [69] Venturini demonstrated that olive oil and fish oil are also protective of oxidative stress in people with metabolic syndrome. [70]

Lipids (fat) are an important macronutrient that our bodies need in order to sustain proper cellular health, cellular energy, vitamin absorption, and hormone production. However, those lipids that are best to consume are nearest to their whole and natural forms. Whole milk from organic, grass-fed animals, butter, and yogurt are good additions to the diet. Eating oily fish like salmon contributes to healthy metabolism and reduces inflammation. Beef can be eaten safely in moderation. So don't be scared to add a little butter or coconut oil to those sautéed mushrooms that are high in vitamin D. That with lipids present allows your body to absorb them!

Lipid or fat in the form of industrialized trans-fatty acid or hydrogenated vegetable has no place in our diet. *None.*

Remove. Replace. Restore.

Remove *all* forms of hydrogenated vegetable oil and industrial TFA. Read the labels on *everything*, especially salad dressing, chips, cookies, and crackers. Remove all "fake butter spreads" from your refrigerator. Kick canola oil, vegetable oil, and shortening out of your baking.

Replace with healthy fats/lipids. For baking or heating, use butter, ghee (clarified butter), lard, and tallow from organic grass-fed sources, or coconut oil. For low heat or salad dressing, use olive oil. Fish oil is fragile, so get it from a reputable source or simply eat it in its whole form from fatty fish like salmon, sardines, or troll-caught tuna. If snacks like crackers and cookies are your downfall, then replace them with crisp green apples or fresh berries.

Restore cardiovascular, metabolic, integumentary, and neurological health. If you are working on restoring metabolic or cardiovascular health, then consult your physician to monitor your blood values while you make dietary changes. Moderation of lipid consumption within a well-balanced diet and activity are the keys. Fat doesn't seem to be all bad as we once thought. In fact, it seems the plasticity of fat works to our benefit. Remember to always listen to your body!

Protein (Not Powder)

> These are isolated nutrients and should be viewed as supplementation sources, not food replacements. If you are capable of eating food, you should eat food.
>
> —Diane Sanfilippo, NC

Protein is considered a macronutrient, like fats and carbohydrates. Protein makes up at least 50% of your body. By definition, protein is a nitrogen-containing macronutrient made from amino acids. Our body needs twenty different amino acids to make all the proteins it requires for:

- structure (tissue, bone, teeth, skin);
- catalysis (enzymatic activity);
- movement (muscles, ligaments, tendons);
- transport (across cell membranes);
- communication (hormones and cell signaling);
- protection (skin, immune system);
- regulation of fluid balance;
- regulation of pH; and
- energy (source of glucose).

Of the twenty amino acids, nine are essential (the body cannot make them or cannot make as much as the body requires). Eleven are nonessential (the body can synthesize these under some conditions, but sometimes they are conditionally essential depending on the circumstances like for optimal growth and development in infants).

Food proteins are categorized as complete (containing all the essential amino acids) or incomplete (lacking or containing very low amounts of one or more essential amino acid). The only food sources of complete amino acid profile are meat, poultry, eggs, and dairy. Plant sources are incomplete and require protein complementation (rice and beans or corn and beans). If avoiding all animal products is part of your lifestyle, then careful assessment and consumption of plant-based proteins is paramount to maintaining health, as is supplementation with a good vitamin B12. Vitamin B12 is primarily in food products from animals, and lack of adequate vitamin B12 can lead to a host of health disruptions.

Lack of adequate amino acids may result in lack of collagen production, difficulty with digestion of nutrients, muscle wasting, anemia or vitamin deficiencies, difficulty coordinating hormonal regulation, weakened immune system, edema and swelling, pH imbalance, and difficulty with blood-sugar regulation. On the flip side, overconsumption of protein and amino acids will lead to fat storage.[3]

One protein that has been well studied in the diabetic population is whey protein from dairy. The diabetic population, those who suffer with metabolic disorders, also have a difficult time healing. Specifically, whey protein has been shown to improve wound healing. [71-76] Whey protein has been linked to decreasing oxidative stress in experimental burn injuries as well.[77]

The benefits of protein extend beyond diabetics into other patient populations. For example, a randomized controlled trial in 2014 found protein-enriched diets (from lean red meat) to be associated with improvements of muscle strength and tissue mass and reducing inflammatory cytokines (IL-6) in elderly women. [78] Even bone marrow cells have been shown to improve skeletal patterning and osteoblast differentiation for craniofacial bone repair and wound healing. [79]

In today's world, there is an onslaught of protein-powder options. There are so many different options, vegetable protein powder, whey protein powder, and many more. Although there is some research that supports the use of whey protein in the diabetic population, I still would caution its use on a regular basis. Here is why. As we discussed earlier, heavily refined and processed foods are actually devoid of most nutrients. One could argue the same goes for protein powder. Supplementing occasionally with a pure protein powder from a natural source (no additives or sugars and known processing) may be necessary with certain conditions, like diabetes or healing. As a regular consumption, it is unnecessary. Should you feel the need to add it to smoothies to dampen the insulin spike for the fruit, then add healthy fat and eat a whole piece of protein instead of protein powder. Probably more important is the purity of the protein powder. Most come with heavy amounts of sugar for taste and selling purposes, which defeats the purpose to begin with. Additionally, unless you find one from a reputable source, organic, non-GMO, grass-fed, then you don't really know what you are getting. There is a place for protein powder occasionally and under certain conditions, but not regularly as meal replacements. Make the green smoothie but forgo the protein powder, and your body will be gaining valuable nutrients.

We need protein and adequate amino acids to provide our bodies the equipment it needs to heal from injury, surgery, or illness. Protein is essential and invaluable in its contribution to our health and recovery.

Remove. Replace. Restore.

Remove inflammatory foods like refined sugar, refined grains, and refined vegetable oil.

Replace with healthy proteins, along with plenty of fruits and vegetables. Whole organic, wild/free-range/grass-fed is always optimal, but not essential. Refined amino acids, as in protein powders, are not always optimal, but they are useful in certain conditions, temporarily. They can be "negative nutrition" in many cases, however. Be sure to always read the label on the protein powder and be sure it is pure and without additives and sugars. Consider including bone broth (see recipe in back) and include long bones for the marrow to aid in healing and recovery.

Restore structure, function, and health by including healthy proteins into a balanced diet, including whole fruits and vegetables, along with adequate exercise and rest.

Carbohydrates (Not Refined)

> The simple answer as to why we get fat is that carbohydrates
> make us so; protein and fat do not.
>
> —Gary Taubes

Carbohydrates are the sugars, fiber, and starch found in plants and tubers (red potato, sweet potato). The carbohydrate provides the body with energy. There are two types, simple carbohydrates and complex carbohydrates. Simple carbohydrates are made up of one or two molecules. Single molecule carbohydrates are called monosaccharides. These are glucose (most abundant in the blood), fructose (from fruits and vegetables), and lactose (from dairy).

The monosaccharaides are, in fact, sugars. The ones to be the most aware of as far as health is concerned are refined sugars and high-fructose corn syrup, but really all caloric sweeteners should get your attention. We discussed these earlier as inflammatory components, and we will address methods to deal with kicking the habit in "Lateral Shift Technique."

The disaccharide is made up of two molecules. These are lactose (most abundant in milk, the one most people are intolerant to), maltose (formed during starch breakdown, important in beer production), and sucrose (most abundant in plants, especially sugar cane and sugar beets). These are still broken down rather easily into single sugars, which are problematic for spiking insulin. However, these are also naturally occurring in many nutrient-rich fruits that have a multitude of vitamins and minerals, which are health promoting. So eating simple carbohydrates in moderation in a balanced nutritional profile is actually health promoting.

Complex carbohydrates consist of many single sugars together with multiple bonds. There are the oligosaccharides that are in many plant foods that make up the cell membrane. Polysaccharides have many single sugars but a different bond, and they are called starches. These foods often are high in fiber, which we are unable to break down, but they act as an intestinal broom as they move through the digestive tract. The complex carbohydrates burn more slowly than simple carbohydrates, providing for more extended energy. A way to slow simple carbohydrate burning down is to add a healthy fat like almond butter.

All plants have carbohydrates. Some have more simple carbohydrates than complex carbohydrates. The sweeter the plant is, the more simple carbohydrates present. Be most cautious of simple carbohydrates, especially refined and processed like high-fructose corn syrup and sweeteners, as they are associated with metabolic disorders[35-37] and impact joint health. [18,80] Eat the rainbow of colors of plants, and you will be improving the nutrient richness of your diet and working on prevention of disease.

Another potential carbohydrate to discuss is alcohol. The question is to drink or not to drink alcohol? I will admit that a nice, quality alcoholic beverage with high-quality alcohol and fresh ingredients is incredibly enjoyable. For example, a fresh mango margarita can't be beat on a hot summer day. From a KISS principle standpoint, it often does not meet the standard criteria of simple. Alcoholic beverages are high calorie, high in simple carbohydrates, and high glycemic loads, and they are absorbed into the bloodstream in the stomach, thereby skipping our natural filtration system in the small intestine. More than that, alcohol is often used as a crutch to deal with something in life that should be honored and dealt with in a more positive way (see chapter 7).

Sometimes it is an easy way to "connect" with people, but I argue that it isn't a true connection, but rather a way to fit in. For me, even a good wine gives me heartburn, but I know a good wine has antioxidants. (Unfortunately many American wines have added colors or sulfites that can be inflammatory.) I have developed a few alternative adult beverages (see "Adult-Friendly Drink Alternative," page 138) that I enjoy, and although I can never call them nutrient-rich, I certainly don't feel depleted afterward as with many other alcoholic beverages. And truly, I always ask myself, "Why do I need to drink right now? Am I anxious? Am I tired? Are my kids driving me crazy? Or is this the only way I know how to be with this person?" Answering yes to any of these scenarios is not a reason to drink. "Or do I simply want a good drink with a good friend to savor this moment?" If it is yes to this question, then I will enjoy.

In the past, though, I would drink to "fit in," because large groups made me a little anxious. Alcoholism runs in my family also, so I have always been on the lookout for it in my life. I have a tendency toward addictive behaviors, and I simply try to choose healthy addictive behaviors. When you find yourself making a habit of wine or alcohol on a daily or weekly basis, then I suggest you look hard at the reason for it.

Working in a hospital taking care of patients, they teach you that if someone says they have five to seven drinks per week, that you should double it for men and triple it for women. Why? Because nobody wants to admit that they drink that much because they inherently know that too much alcohol isn't good for you or your *liver*.

In fact, recent research demonstrates that fatty liver disease that was once thought to be purely due to alcoholism is, in fact, now popping up in young kids. Why? Because alcohol is excessive in sugar and sometimes toxins, which results in fatty deposits in the liver. So is soda, with its high sugar content and chemicals. Both are caused by sugar. One simple sugar is high-fructose corn syrup, and the other is sugar alcohol. Both have chemicals and additives that are an additional burden to the body.

Carbohydrates are necessary and critical to cellular energy for your body and brain. To remove all carbohydrates would lead to severe fatigue.

Eating complex carbohydrates gives you maximal health benefits and energy, and simple carbohydrates spike blood sugar levels, often leaving you craving more and low on energy.

Remove. Replace. Restore.

Remove all refined sugars and flours, as they are high concentrations of sugar that will spike the body's insulin, leading to an inflammatory response.

Replace with whole, organic fruits and vegetables for a treat. Add a healthy fat like almond butter or sunflower-seed butter for a slow energy burn.

Restore cellular energy and health.

Healing

> The natural healing force within each of us is the greatest force in getting well.
>
> —Hippocrates

The capacity of your body to heal in many cases is limitless. Our limits in healing are often products of our own self-doubt or even the doubt of authority figures or health care providers. For me, even just five years ago, I would never have believed most of what I share with you today. That alone didn't make the information untrue. One of the goals of this book is to provide adequate evidence to support the lifestyle recommendations. The only person who has to believe in it is you in order for you to be willing to make adjustments in your life. However, if you do have a medical condition, the other person from whom you need support (or belief that nutrition can help healing) is your physician. Oftentimes, having the research or data to support you may help your physician better support you as you seek health. Let me share another story with you.

I personally had this experience with my father-in-law and his neurologist at the Veterans Administration (VA). After my husband and I made those changes to his diet and he was doing well, we both agreed that depression was playing a role in his decline. From our clinical experience, a temporary or long-term solution to assist in getting him back on track was to address the depression with medication so that he could work on eating better and moving more. Parkinson's disease is a devastating progressive autoimmune disease, and anyone who has experienced it would agree that depression is often something you need to look out for. Up until this point, almost every single patient with Parkinson's disease I have ever worked with has been on an antidepressant. I am not necessarily a proponent of it per se, but it is a tool. Our goal was to support him to then start working on the KISS principles so that he potentially could remove many of his medications.

I took a day off work to go with my father-in-law for his neurologist appointment. When we spoke with the doctor, the doctor looked at me and said, "I never see people with Parkinson's disease suffer with depression." I couldn't believe it. He refused to prescribe him the medications. I will never know for sure if the doctor's response was because he didn't believe how bad my father-in-law was, if he didn't believe how good my father-in-law got with nutrition and exercise, or maybe he really hadn't seen a Parkinson's patient with depression before. Either way, I was not prepared with the information about the links between depression and Parkinson's disease to argue with him. It was a hard lesson for me to learn. I realized, though, that without the support of his doctor in addressing the depression, nutrition, and lifestyle, there would be *no* change for my father-in-law.

More to the point, as the patient or the consumer, you need information and information you can share with your physicians. They may or may not have time or experience in the new information you bring. Maybe if I had done my homework, then I could have brought a few articles, books, or resources with me to validate my concern. The details on what affect certain food, or food-like substances, or medications potentially have on your body are supported by research.

The best news of all is that even if you find yourself sick from your past exposures, there is opportunity to heal. There are certain diseases that may have limited recovery, but the likelihood of better control and improvement is with good nutrition.

We discussed many food components that have the potential to cause inflammation in table 4. Below, table 5 is nutritional components that support healing, enhance anti-inflammatory mechanisms, or both. In fact, there are many more healing nutritional components than inflammatory.

Beneficial Dietary Component	Food in which Found	Healing or anti-inflammatory response
Probiotics[7,62,63,81,82]	Naturally fermented vegetables and dairy (pickles, sauerkraut, kimchi, yogurt, kefir)	Improved gastrointestinal function, manufacture vitamins, anti-inflammatory, Increase nutrient absorption, prevent infection, digest lactose
Prebiotics[81]	Resistant starch (potato, plantain, inulin)	Anti-inflammatory
Leucine-rich diet[83]	Eggs, spirulina, cheese, beef, pork	Improve tendon strength
Olive oil[84,85]	100% pure, cold-pressed olive oil	Decrease stress response, improve glycogen response in liver
Aloe vera[86]	Aloe vera (juice or capsules)	Improves wound healing
Gelatin/collagen[79,86,87]	Pure gelatin or collagen hydrolysate, bone broth	Antioxidant effects
Chinese herbal formula (Sini Tang)[88]	(Recommend consultation with an herbalist)	Anti-inflammatory for heart
Antioxidants[89-94]	Anthocyanins (Blue, red and purple berries, cherries, purple grapes, red cabbage), betalains (beets, cactus)	Anti-inflammatory for tendons, reduce oxidative stress, antiaging, improves lungs
Biotin[95]	Green leafy vegetables, liver	Decrease inflammation

Bovine colostrum[96]	Bovine colostrum	Reduces gut damage from NSAIDS
Brazil nuts[97]	Brazil nuts	Decreases inflammation
Green coffee bean extract (Chlorogenic acid)[98]	Green coffee bean extract, prunes	Decreases protein cross linking
Resveratrol[99-104]	Purple grapes, bilberries, blueberries	Improves muscle function, anti-inflammatory, joint protection
Curcumin (turmeric)[105-107]	Turmeric	Anti-inflammatory, joint protection
Docosahexaenoic acid (DHA)[56,108-118]	Oily fish (salmon, tuna, sardines, mackerel, and trout)	Neuroplasticity, anti-inflammatory, joint protection, improve dopamine neurons
Cocoa[119,120]	100% chocolate	Anti-inflammatory, anti-oxidant
Glycosaminoglycan (Glucosamine)[121,122]	Glucosamine/chondroitin sulfate supplements	Decrease inflammation of gut lining, regulates cellular death
Vitamin D[123-127]	Liver, grass-fed dairy, fermented cod liver oil, fish, portabella mushrooms, egg yolk, sunshine	Tendon strength, joint health, decrease risk of autoimmune disease, improved stroke recovery
Spirulina[119,128]	Spirulina, raw or dried	Stem cell proliferation, health protection

Lean red meat[78]	Lean red meat; beef, wild game	Improve muscle strength and healing
Vitamin C[34,129,130]	Citrus, peppers, kale	Improve tendon mobility, antioxidant
Whey protein [71-74,77]	Whey protein powder	Improves wound healing, especially if diabetic
Conjugated and alpha linoleic acid[131]	Grass-fed/pasture-raised dairy cream	Improves metabolic health and strengthens gut barrier
High-fat dairy[132]	Whole milk	Anti-inflammatory activity especially if have metabolic disorder
Vitamin E[129]	Nuts (almonds, hazelnuts, pine nuts), nut oils	Antioxidant
Yeast hydrolysate[133]	Yeast extract	Joint health

Table 5: Nutritional components found to support healing, anti-inflammatory mechanisms, or both and the whole foods in which they occur. Above referenced foods can be found on government website http://ndb.nal.usda.gov/.

What is most amazing to me is the fact that simple foods like green leafy vegetables, nuts/seeds, berries, and healthy protein can help you heal and fight disease. That is pretty amazing, and simple. Even if you are unfortunate enough to suffer a stroke and have a metabolic disorder, your potential for rehabilitation and functional recovery potential improves when you improve your systemic inflammatory status. [23] One way to improve your inflammatory state is to eat anti-inflammatory and nutrient-rich whole foods.

I would add that if you are recovering from an injury, illness, leaky gut, surgery, or even postpartum vaginal or C-section delivery and you have all your whole foods nutrition in check, then you may want to consider a traditional addition of bone broth and vegetable broth (recipe in the back). Those are both ways to get bioavailable vitamins, minerals like potassium and calcium, and vitamins A and C. The key to these preparations is quality bone, including long bones from grass-fed organic beef, and patience. Bone broth is another way to increase calcium, collagen, gelatin, and marrow. All components help with healing of soft tissue and ligaments. I personally make bone broth on a regular basis and freeze it, so I use it regularly in cooking, but I also have it on hand for when I sense a viral cold starting.

As anecdotal evidence of the power of bone broth, let me share a story. A dear friend of mine, Jared, started to include bone broth in his daily routine as he recovered from brain surgery and chemotherapy. The doctors were monitoring his white blood cell count as a measure of how well his body was doing. At one point, his levels were a little low. He started drinking bone broth daily for seven days, and he had his white blood cell counted again. It had risen by one hundred points. We will never know for sure if it had only to do with the bone broth, except that bone broth was the only thing he specifically changed. Jared was pretty excited to see a measurable change.

It is important to note that none of these recommendations are to take place entirely of traditional medical care. There is a time and a place when medication is needed. Following surgery is a good time to take an antibiotic to prevent infection, but you may find that eating well and moving may keep your pain at a level that doesn't require pain medication. And supplementing with a good professional probiotic may be warranted to support the gut. Absolutely talk with your health care provider to make a good plan.

If you are at a standstill in the healing processs, then you may want to consider supplementation, especially if you are trying to heal a leaky gut. I will not recommend a blanket supplement or multivitamin or mineral. There is debate about whether or not they are necessary. However, should your family history or medical history dictate that you are at risk for a certain disease, then I would consider vitamin and mineral supplementation. Given our family history of Parkinson's disease and Alzheimer's disease, we do take a multivitamin/mineral supplement along with fish oil to reach the optimum daily intake (ODI) as described in the "Nutrient Deficiency" section.

There is concern that our food today is not as nutrient-rich as it used to be, given our farming practices and nutrient-depleted soil. It is true. Buying locally and organically will help maximize nutrient density. If you have illness, you are likely nutrient deficient somewhere, and it's likely that if you address it first by switching to whole nutrient-rich foods and avoiding depleting foods, your body will begin to restore health.

No supplement can improve a bad diet. A supplement is meant to be just that, a means to enhance an already healthy diet. Often patients continue with heavy alcohol consumption on a daily basis and even use it as a meal replacement, and then wonder why they have pain, don't heal, are always sick, and don't feel well. In response to the degradation, they turn to a host of supplements. Yet they still don't recover.

You must be careful where the supplements come from too, because that is another source of potential gut irritation. Are they made from natural sources? Are they organic? Are they synthetic? What else is in the supplement that may be potentially harmful to your gut? You see how complicated this gets. The whole point is to live by simple principles, and supplements may be a source of complication when simply eating whole foods and avoiding inflammatory foods as described above are the safest ways to health and wellness.

If you are stuck, it is always best to seek help. There are many health care providers that are available and up to date on how to use whole foods nutrition and appropriate supplementation to support healing, and even some medical doctors are starting to come along. A place to start would be looking for a functional medicine professional, specially trained dieticians, or nutritionists, holistic health providers like acupuncturists, and even specially trained physical therapists if you have a painful condition. Understand that medical treatment is great at keeping you alive and should not be avoided, but holistic health providers can help improve the quality of life and supplement traditional care. These alternative or holistic health care providers can help bridge the gap between body systems as they work with the whole body and systems together, not in isolation.

Remove. Replace. Restore.

Remove inflammatory foods, refined sugar, refined grains, refined vegetable oils, and even alcohol. (Sorry, but to heal, you need to.)

Replace with whole, organic, non-GMO produce, grass-fed meats, wild-caught fish, healthy fats, bone broth, and mineral broth.

Restore health, prevent disease, or manage your disease better.

Back to the Basics; Traditional

> You don't have to cook fancy or complicated masterpieces—just good food from fresh ingredients.
>
> —Julia Child

Separately, all of this information seems a bit complicated. Together, it is quite simple. There are new food guidelines lined out for us by the government in the shape of a plate. The plate includes fruits, vegetables, grains, protein, and milk. But some have offered up a more simple solution to the "MyPlate." You need to eat plants and animals and drink *water*. The ratios depend on your lifestyle, activity level, age, and medical conditions. Here are some samples of what your dinner plate should look like:

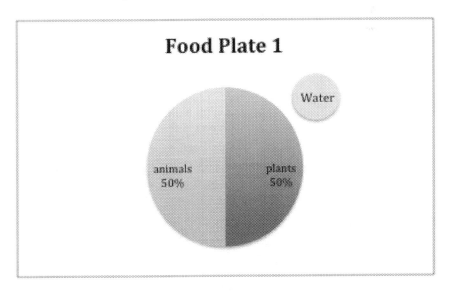

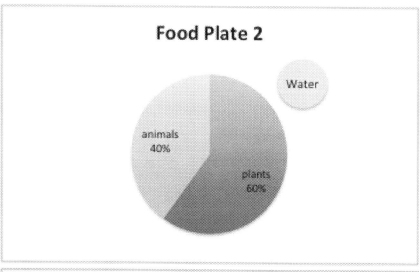

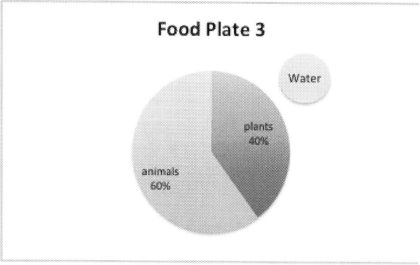

Each section should be filled with a whole food, not something that looks like food. And getting back to the basics in cooking is important and simple. If you purchase quality whole ingredients, then simply cooking it until its ready with some salt and pepper is enough. For example, a pan-seared grass-fed steak with a side of sautéed mushrooms and a green salad would be a great meal for breakfast, lunch, or dinner. In my household, we say, "Dinner, it's what's for breakfast."

You always want a mix of raw and cooked vegetables. I always have a supply of fresh greens, carrots, and fresh fruit in the refrigerator for any-time-of-day snack or meal-on-the-go. Most of what you eat should need only be washed and cut. If it comes in a box, look at the ingredients extremely carefully. If you couldn't make it on your own, you probably shouldn't eat it.

I would like to share a few more thoughts on grains. We discussed earlier the detrimental health effects of gluten-containing grains as well as refined grains being equated to sugar. Additionally, grains are often treated with pesticide and are a GMO product. If having grains is an important part of your life, be sure to purchase organic and non-GMO, rinse before you prepare, and even ferment or sprout before cooking. This traditional preparation will decrease the phytic acid content so that you won't have competition with binding nutrients, thereby decreasing the potential for inflammation. Keep in mind that brown rice has a lower glycemic load (less spiking of the blood glucose) than does white rice. Enjoying these naturally gluten-free grains with a healthy fat like butter to slow the absorption and even adding nutrients, like making it with a mineral-rich bone broth, would be more nutritious.

Another traditional process is called fermentation. This process allows preservation of food while maintaining if not improving nutrient richness. There are many books on home fermentation that would be worth looking into, but maybe a little later in your journey.

Some simple meal ideas:

- Baked chicken breast with olive oil, salt, pepper, and lemon, with steamed broccoli and a fresh green salad with homemade vinaigrette
- Pan-seared, grass-fed beefsteak with sautéed mushrooms and green salad
- Ground grass-fed beef, pan-fried, with lettuce wraps, sliced tomato, onion, and avocado, with baked sweet potato and a green salad

In addition to *what* is for dinner, *who* prepares dinner is important. I have heard it said, "Everyone belongs in the kitchen." If everyone eats dinner together, everyone should play a role, no matter how minimal, in preparing the meal. At our home, my youngest sometimes washes the carrots. My older boys sometimes scramble the eggs for breakfast. My husband will barbecue the meat when he is available. The point is that food preparation and eating is a family affair. The burden of meal prep should not fall on any single person when part of a family. This may seem idealistic, I know. Yet we all need to eat food to live, so we all should be in the kitchen participating. It is a great opportunity for learning, for connection, and even for fun.

Remove. Replace. Restore.
Remove complicated packaged foods.
Replace with simple, whole ingredients. Good, wholesome ingredients do not need much prep to taste good.
Restore family mealtime, together.

Lateral Shift Technique

> I can't change the direction of the wind, but I can adjust my sails to always reach my destination.
>
> —Jimmy Dean

Depending on where you are in your life, you may or may not have developed a sweet tooth. For me, with my history as an athlete in the 1990s, I lived heavily on high-processed carbs (pasta, bread, pizza, etc.) and refined sugar (Gatorade, candy bars, ice cream, etc.). Weight management was not my problem, but the high-sugar diet has left me with lots of habits and cravings. Over time, eating a whole foods–inspired diet has improved it. In order to correct the sweet tooth, I used the "lateral shift" technique to get control. Let me introduce you to the lateral shift technique.

In mechanical diagnosis and treatment (MDT) terms, the lateral shift is used to describe spinal deformities when the hips and shoulders are not in line. Shoulders are often shifted over to one side making you look crooked. This is generally an indication that you need a manual mechanical correction to essentially get straightened out. The lateral shift generally has a negative connotation. But correcting it allows you to become straightened out. Now let's look at the positive lateral shift correction as it relates to sugar.

I use this term, lateral shift, to help those who struggle with sugar cravings. As we have discussed the many negative health problems associated with added refined sugars in many forms, I'd like to emphasize that natural sugars that occur in whole form, like those in fruits and vegetables, are, in fact, healthy.

So when the urge for something sweet strikes, perform the lateral shift technique! Take that urge and simply move over to a banana or sliced green apple paired with some almond butter to slow glucose absorption, or grab a small handful of fresh organic blueberries or raspberries. The fructose in these items in their whole form make the fruit sweet, but the fruits also have added fiber, vitamins, and antioxidants that fight off illness and support health. Pair these with some healthy fats, and you also slow the absorption of the fructose to keep from spiking your blood sugar.

In fact, a prospective cohort study of over seventy-five thousand nurses in 2000 demonstrated that eating carbohydrates with a low glycemic index (GI is a measurement to determine how the food impacts your blood sugar) was actually associated with a decrease in risk of coronary heart disease. Low glycemic foods include *fruit*! On the other hand, consuming high glycemic index foods (refined grains, refined sugars) resulted in an increased risk of developing coronary heart disease.[134]

Some fruits that have a low glycemic index:

- Apples
- Bananas (the less ripe ones)
- Blueberries
- Cranberries
- Grapefruit
- Grapes
- Kiwi
- Lemons
- Oranges
- Plums
- Prunes

- Raspberries
- Strawberries

Be sure to avoid high glycemic index foods:

- White potatoes (especially chips)
- Refined grains
- Refined sugar
- Cookies
- Baked goods
- Alcohol

For a more exhaustive description and lists, please check out the World's Healthiest Foods website: www.whfoods.com.

I personally find living sugar-free is more difficult than gluten-free. Almost everything has a sweetener in it, unfortunately. By eating whole foods, you will already be improving the sugar cravings. Some techniques that help to curb the sweet tooth are:

- eating protein and healthy fat with every meal to keep the blood sugar spikes from occurring;
- planning ahead for when you will be out of the home for extended periods of time, having readily available snacks on hand to help curb your hunger and improve your self-control; and
- eating only quality sugar. (Don't just eat any candy bar; eat the 75% organic cocoa chocolate that is sweetened with raw honey or maple syrup. Don't waste a good treat on a Snickers bar that is so unsatisfying.)

There are some other fun options of lateral shift recipes in the back of the book to enjoy occasionally. No matter, when the sweet tooth hits, grab an apple or raspberries. If you are really working on weight loss at this point in your life, then you may need to be more restrictive, but truly this book is about lifestyle habits that are sustainable, and removing the joy of eating is problematic for me. The more you fill in with healthy, nutritious *whole* foods, the less space there is for junk. So keep crowding out the junk food.

Remove. Replace. Restore.

Remove high-glycemic foods like refined grains, refined sugar, processed foods, alcohol, and other nutrient-depleting foods.

Replace with low-glycemic foods like whole fruits and vegetables and healthy protein and fat. Use the lateral shift technique whenever the sweet tooth hits. Become a sugar snob. Over time, the cravings will diminish, and you will notice the sweetness of a raw carrot!

Restore blood sugar regulation and enjoy the health benefits of added nutrients to your diet with the natural sweetness of whole, fresh organic fruits and vegetables.

Soaring Tips

Eating whole nutritious food is a basic principle. It is as simple as it gets for sustaining and even improving health. Yet it is surprisingly difficult to achieve in today's world. Here are a few challenges I have noticed and how our family addresses them.

School time is a battle to keep the sugar-sweetened drinks, snacks, and cakes in check. I find that if you bring a box of "better" treats that can be stored for those times, all of our teachers have been very cooperative. In fact, the teachers have been extremely supportive, as they know that our kids' classroom learning is much better when they eat nutritious whole foods over Goldfish crackers or "sugar tubes" called yogurt. Simply put, keep your meals for kids at school looking like the meals at home. Keep open communication with your children's teachers, but learning to live with the exposure to unhealthy food is an important skill for your kids to develop at a young age.

Children's sporting events are another challenge. You would be surprised how much sugar is consumed, despite the children wanting to optimize their performance. We always come prepared, but more interestingly, since we eat whole foods, generally our kids aren't even interested in sugar snacks because they know how the sugar makes them feel. I have included a recipe for "SOAR Spa Water" and "SOAR Spritzer" for those days when you do actually need to replenish minerals. Even the International Society of Sports Nutrition (ISSN) has an official stand on energy drinks like Gatorade. They outline nine different points that mention that the ingredients in energy shots and energy drinks are not proven beneficial, and even recommend further study to demonstrate their safety. They further state that athletes should consider the potential impact of these high-glycemic drinks on metabolic health and that caffeine may negatively impact motor-skill performance. The ISSN recommends athletes with preexisting health conditions should avoid these drinks altogether. [135] Cheers to ISSN for taking a very well thought-out stance. I applaud them. I hope someday that local Little Leagues will take note of the ISSN recommendations so that the concession stands for children's events will host more nutritious snacks and refreshments.

I would argue that five-year-old athletes playing T-ball do not need any extra replenishing of calories to stand around, but maybe ten-year-old athletes during a ninety-minute soccer game do. Again, we simply plan ahead. I always have fresh fruits and vegetables on hand to grab and go. What is wrong with actually pealing and eating a whole orange after the game? Bribing the children to play hard with things like promises of sugary drinks afterward is extremely complicated for not only health, but also mental well-being. I refuse to bribe my kids to play sports. If they don't want to play because they aren't allowed sugary treats or they lose their temper due to hunger, then we need to understand better the underlying problem, and it is *not* because they are dying of hunger.

Booby traps are another thing to be aware of. They really are everywhere. It is food-industry marketing. With the fad of paleo diet, there are things marked "paleo" or "caveman" or "gluten-free" or "no high-fructose corn syrup." They are marketing to the eye, so that you might forget to look at the ingredients to see what is actually in the food item. Never buy anything based on the label on the front, except whole fruits and vegetable with the USDA-regulated "organic" and "non-GMO" labels. Trust no one. Make a habit of reading *all* labels. Once you start, you will realize how much marketing goes into selling food.

I didn't even mention how the grocery store puts the "healthy" fruit right at the entrance and then places the chips toward the checkout. Marketing studies have shown that if you buy healthy first, you are more likely to spend more money on other junk in the store, especially if you are a mother. So for me the blinders are off, and I fall less frequently to the marketing schemes. Yet I am not perfect.

Another helpful tool for a busy lifestyle is using premade meals. There are some local sources of healthy premade meals that can be delivered, and some companies ship to the home nationwide. For me, this is an invaluable resource. It is simply impossible to be home cooking a meal and at soccer practice at the same time. So we do use these premade meal options during those times. As eating whole foods becomes more and more popular, these resources are more readily available. I also enjoy knowing that the chef cooking the meals is concerned about quality of the ingredients, so I feel relieved that even my form of "fast food" is still healthy food. There are even better food options out there for frozen premade meals; you just have to look at the ingredients.

More and more restaurants have gluten-free menus, and some even have non-GMO products. When in doubt, eating out, always ask for what you want. The reality is you went out to be served what you want without the effort, so don't be shy. Please be kind and courteous and tip appropriately, but most establishments want business to keep coming back. One idea is to get a hamburger with lettuce wrap, sometimes called "protein style," and a side of veggies or side salad instead of fries.

Perfection in eating is not the answer. The answer is eating to fuel your body. Most of what we eat today does not fuel our body but depletes it. Giving up entire food groups (like dairy, grains, or legumes) causes many people to struggle. Yet if you feel so tied to something that you feel like you can't give it up, maybe that is an indication that you actually need to—at least for a while. It may not be for a lifetime, but start with thirty days. You won't know how your body feels without it unless you remove it for a minimum of thirty days and then reintroduce it. Personally, I have found a balance with dairy in its best form from cows and an even better relationship with dairy from smaller animals like goat or sheep because they have a much lower lactose concentration. Fermented cow's milk in the form of Parmesan cheese is ok for me since the length of time the fermentation occurs allows for near complete breakdown of the lactose. Legumes are an occasional treat in the form of fermented organic soy sauce or organic black beans. Truly, "occasional" means once a month, maybe. I occasionally include gluten-free, non-GMO and organic grains in whole form, prepared traditionally.

The point with all of this is that your personal needs may be slightly different than mine, yet the principle of eating well and eating whole food absolutely is the same for all of us across all ages.

Remove. Replace. Restore.

Remove refined sugars, refined grains, refined vegetable oils, and refined and processed food or drink.

Replace with whole organic and non-GMO produce, wild/grass-fed/organic meats and seafood, and plenty of *fresh* water.

Restore health, well-being, and prevent disease.

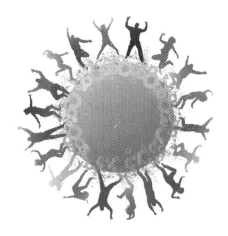

CHAPTER 3: MOVE WELL

Life requires movement.

—Aristotle

What Is Movement?

Movement is defined as an act of changing physical location or position. For me as a physical therapist, the movement you do throughout the day *must* include full range of motion of the joints. Our standard American life tends toward spine flexion in the form of sitting in front of a computer, in a car, on a couch watching TV, and lifting, which is all flexion. It is not that sitting alone is a problem as much as chronic sitting means you are not moving your joints through their full range of motion.

A healthy joint is a flexible joint. When you stop moving joints, the tendency is for them to get stiff, soft tissue shortens, and you lose range of motion. Once the motion is lost, the strength of the muscle supporting that joint begins to weaken. It is a vicious cycle.

Healthy movements may include a full squat. A full squat from start to finish allows the hip, knees, and ankles to go through a near full range of motion. Performing a cobra maneuver on the ground can allow a near full extension of the ankles, knees, hip, spine, and wrists. A relaxing prayer stretch allows full unloaded shoulders, knees, ankles, and spine flexion. By adding in a few other motions like spinal rotation and wrist flexion, you have nearly covered all the joints in just a few moments. Performing some of these exercises regularly throughout the day, should you need to sit, is a great way to keep the joints healthy, lubricated, and flexible.

Some good basic foundational flexibility exercises (See appendix 6 for photos of below exercises):

Extension in lying with neck extension
Downward dog, calf and hamstring stretching, knees bent
Prayer stretch
Kneeling shoulder extension stretch
Kneeling shoulder internal rotation stretch
Kneeling cervical rotation
Kneeling cervical side bending
Lumbar rotation in lying
Hip external rotation

Remove. Replace. Restore.
Remove immobility.
Replace with simple whole body movements to maintain joint integrity. A daily regimen is best.
Restore joint health.

The Best Exercise

The best exercise is the one that you will do.

—Grant Glass, PT

I often get asked about what is the best exercise routine. It is confusing with all the exercise fads out there. There is CrossFit, Kaia FIT, P90X, Zumba, yoga, Insanity, kettlebell, and many more. The real answer is, as Grant Glass put it, the best exercise is the best exercise for you. My best exercise is different from yours. Anything that gets you moving regularly is what is best. The exercise needs to fit your body, your lifestyle, and your needs.

A good exercise will provide you with cardiovascular training, weight-bearing (to build and keep your bones strong), and resistance to build muscle strength. All of the above exercise fads do provide for most of those components. A simple exercise program will often improve disability, function, quality of life, decrease painful status, [136] improve antioxidant (antiaging) enzymes, [137] stimulate neuroplasticity (the ability to learn and adapt), [138] improve subjective well-being, [139] increase volume of white and gray matter in the brain, [140] and increase stress resistance, [138] just to name a few of the positive effects.

Some good basic foundational strengthening exercises (See appendix 7 for photos of below exercises.):

Squats
Lunges
Push-ups
Planks front
Planks side
Heel raises
Walking

What happens when you can't move because of pain or flexibility problems? Seek help from a movement specialist. I am biased here, but a good physical therapist is one of the best resources. I recommend finding one who has not only PT after his or her name, but other letters like "Cert MDT" or "OCS," since it means they care about continued learning to provide the best care for their patients.

Remove. Replace. Restore.

Remove stagnancy.

Replace with an exercise routine that fits your lifestyle, personality and goals.

Restore a sense of well-being and overall health.

Don't Beat Yourself Up

If you can't fly, then run,
if you can't run, then walk,
if you can't walk, then crawl,
but whatever you do,
you have to keep moving forward.

—Martin Luther King Jr

Probably the biggest hurdle with fad exercise routines is the shaming that goes on when you do not do it absolutely every day. I have a few reasons this bothers me from a physical therapy perspective. First, I don't believe in shaming policies; they make some people feel badly about themselves. Shaming is a great way to get a quick result and even makes a fair amount of money. Second, there is such a thing as too much exercise. Sense of well-being does *not* get better with more frequent, greater intensity and duration of exercise compared to moderate intensity. [139] High-intensity exercise five to seven days a week actually sets you up for injury as well as adrenal fatigue.

Yet where is the balance? What is enough, and what is too little? I agree with most, that our Western culture is relatively physically inactive, yet I do not believe high-intensity exercise alone is actually healthful. The science on the perfect answer is evolving, but either way, only you can know what is best for you. A study even challenged the World Health Organizations recommendation as too much for physical health. The World Health Organization recommends the below:

- Five- to seventeen-year-olds should accumulate at least sixty minutes of moderate to vigorous intensity physical activity daily.
- Eighteen- to sixty-year-old and older adults should do at least one hundred and fifty minutes of moderate-intensity aerobic physical activity throughout the week or at least seventy-five minutes of vigorous-intensity aerobic physical activity throughout the week or an equivalent.

A research article demonstrates that the more minutes spent performing vigorous intensity activity significantly reduces the level of subjective well-being. [139] Another confirms that exercise much less than recommended current guidelines was associated with lower mortality. [141] For me, I have found that as a married, working mother of three kids, it feels nearly impossible to meet this expectation without losing sleep, losing time to prepare healthy meals, losing time with my family, or simply losing my mind. Many of the home programs are moderate to vigorous activity five to six days per week anywhere from thirty to sixty minutes. That is a total of one hundred fifty to three hundred minutes per week. Not to mention, that this number doesn't include any of the functional movements and activities required for living an active life.

I have tried to keep up those levels of activity and even tried to recommend them to my patients. Yet everyone fails. Why? Because it just isn't sustainable; it's too hard. Not to mention if you live a busy work or home life, aren't you getting lots of activity walking up and down the stairs, lifting groceries, walking across soccer fields? I have settled in on working out twice per week for vigorous exercise that totals maybe thirty to sixty minutes, and then I live my daily life. If I can get a nice hike in or walking with a friend, then I get a bonus. I move my body every day with a few simple movements that incorporate flexibility and strengthening, but I don't consider them moderate exercise even.

In order to keep up a significantly vigorous level of exercise, like a college athlete, then you *must* have your whole foods nutrition dialed in, without a doubt. Excessive carbohydrate loading in the form of processed and refined carbs or even protein shakes or energy drinks still will potentially set you up for joint disorders, healing problems, metabolic disorders, and even autoimmune disease in the future. It is possible to live even a life of daily vigorous exercise so long as careful planning of the other KISS principles are taken into account. Even the best of athletes take time off from rigorous activity. For me, I want to simply be healthy and live a long life with my family. My personal goal is not to be a fitness model, just a healthy role model for my children and my patients.

Remove. Replace. Restore.
Remove shaming policies and guilt driven motivators.

Replace with simple, healthy movement that feels the best for you and your lifestyle and goals.

Restore health and a sense of well-being.

Sitting Is Sickness, or Is Movement Health?

Nothing happens until something moves.

—Albert Einstein

In the world of physical therapy, we were trained throughout school that sitting slouched was the absolute worst-case scenario for your spine. Your spine would degenerate, which could result in chronic pain. Therapists worked diligently to retrain people to sit with normal lumbar curve (lordosis) to prevent this inevitable degradation of the spine. Then something funny happened: people stopped being able to flex their spines. In mechanical diagnosis and treatment, that is classified as a flexion dysfunction, meaning that the tissue around the joints shortened and remodeled to disallow flexion. So losing flexion range of motion isn't good either, right?

My newfound perspective on sitting is that it is a normal movement we should do sometimes, even daily. We were neither designed to stand and walk all day, every day, nor were we designed to sit in a chair all day, every day. And what would happen if we sat on the ground? Can you imagine sitting on the ground? Maybe you haven't in a long time. But it is good practice because being able to get up from the ground is a good predictor of health.[142]

Sitting becomes unhealthy when we remain sitting in one spot for extended periods of time. Yet there are jobs that require computer work for many hours of the day. I believe that it isn't sitting itself that begets illness as much as the absence of movement. Movement is what our bodies strive for. Even in the hospital on bedrest you lose one-third of your muscle strength for every day you don't move. That is why you always want physical therapy ordered as soon as possible to prevent degradation. I digress a bit, but the point is this: if your job requires sitting for extended periods of time, find a way to incorporate movement. Sitting less and moving more is associated with improved health. [141] There have even been studies done on treadmill-desk use or adjusting desks that allow movement, both having benefits in reducing metabolic-risk biomarkers. [143]

Here are a few suggestions to incorporate more movement if you have a job that requires sitting from the cheapest to the most expensive:

1. Set a timer for every hour to stand up and perform a few quick stretches like extension in standing, extension in lying with full neck extension (appendix 6, image 16), walking around your chair, or performing a few squats (image 6 and appendix 7, image 28).

2. Use a foam roller to reverse the thoracic kyphosis (images 7 and 8).

3. Try a therapy ball chair with or without the stand that allows pelvic movement and weight shifting (image 9). A DynaDisc on top of a standard chair works similarly (image 10).

4. Purchase an adjustable-height desk surface that allows elevating and lowering easily to alternate between sitting and standing. If you were able to use a laptop and set up a low and high working surface, then that would work also.

5. Purchase a tread desk that fits overtop a treadmill that allows for low walking speeds while working.

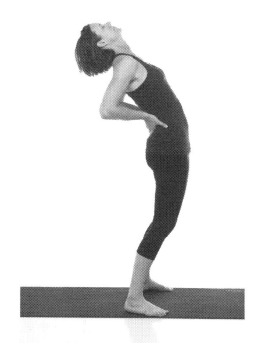

Extension in standing

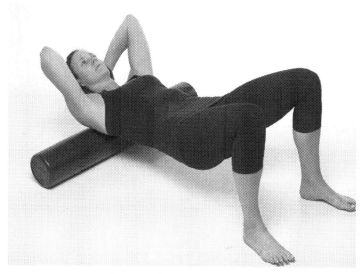

Foam roller curve reversal

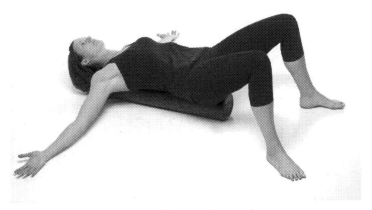

Foam roller angel stretch

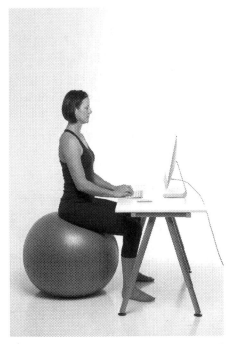

Proper dynamic sitting on a gym ball

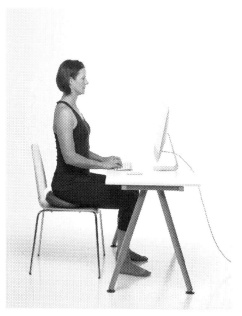

Proper dynamic sitting on a DynaDisc

What is too much sitting? That is a difficult question to answer. From an evolutionary perspective, we took breaks from vigorous hunting and gathering, but even in our resting, we changed our positions frequently. We never sat completely still for hours on end. Recent discussions among health care researchers indicated concerns about sitting greater than five to seven hours/day leading to an increase in mortality (or increase potential rate of death). A recent cross-sectional and ten-year prospective study that was presented in poster form from the Canadian Multicenter Osteoporosis Study (www.camos.org) found that even the sedentary behavior of sitting more than five to seven hours/day was not related to increased mortality if movement was included regularly. [144] Although the study was self-reported data, it still is meaningful. It may not be that sitting is the problem so much unless sitting means you are not moving. The above recommendations can help optimize movement even while sitting. Demonizing sitting gives us the wrong focus, while optimizing movement even in sitting is better.

Remove. Replace. Restore.
Remove stagnant postures and demonizing any single position.

Replace with simple movements, regularly throughout the day. Sit on the floor and get up.

Restore spinal health.

Nutrient Deficiency

A flower cannot blossom without sunshine, and man cannot live without love.

—Max Muller

How is nutrient deficiency related to movement and not eating? Well, the answer will become obvious. Nutrient deficiencies as they relate to how we eat are simply a given. Our food processing and farming practices today render our food less nutritious than it used to be. Healthy eating, possibly with vitamin and mineral supplementation, is a good way to support the body for those deficits. However, there are two vitamins and minerals that I would like to focus on as they relate to movement—vitamin D and calcium.

As a physical therapist, many of my patients have arthritic disease of the joints. During my traditional training, I received minimal education related to the importance of vitamin D and calcium, except that they are important for bone strength, and deficits are in part what lead to osteoporosis (thinning of the bones). However, I am interested in what role vitamin D and calcium play in arthritic conditions and if there is a link to joint health and vitamin D and calcium. And so I have done more research.

First, let's look at these two separately for what they each do, where they come from, and what happens if you don't have enough.

Vitamin D, specifically vitamin D3 in it most natural form, is synthesized from cholesterol in the presence of sunlight. Without sunlight, the body does not produce vitamin D. Vitamin D is necessary for calcium absorption, which means it operates more like a hormone than a true vitamin. Vitamin D comes in limited amounts in food sources. The richest sources outside of sunshine of vitamin D are butterfat, eggs, liver, organ meats, marine oils, and seafood like shrimp and crab. [145] Deficiency of vitamin D has been linked to osteopenia (bone loss), osteoporosis (severe bone loss resulting often in fracture), cancer, type 1 diabetes, multiple sclerosis, and even cardiovascular disease. [126,146] In

71

addition to these diseases, vitamin D deficiency has been linked to many other disease like early inflammatory arthritis (a precursor to rheumatoid arthritis), [147] osteoarthritis of the knee, [125] and autoimmune disease like systemic lupus erythematous (SLE), rheumatoid arthritis (RA), and type 2 diabetes (T2DM). [148] Vitamin D status can even be used as a predictor of prognosis for patients with acute ischemic stroke. [127] Vitamin D is clearly not only important for bone strength but also joint health, metabolic health, and even brain health.

Calcium is a mineral that is readily available in dairy products including cheese, milk and yogurt and bone broth (especially broth made with long marrow bones). In these forms, the calcium is most readily absorbable. The calcium available in meats, vegetables, and grains is difficult to absorb due to presence of iron and zinc. The phytic acid present in grains, if not properly soaked, fermented, and sprouted, will bind the calcium, making it less available for absorption. Deficiency of calcium has been linked to hypertension (high blood pressure), colon cancer, osteoporosis, osteomalacia, and rickets.[146]

Vitamin D *and* calcium work together to produce strong bones and teeth and normal growth. Without calcium, vitamin D cannot absorb the vital ingredient for strong bones. Without vitamin D, calcium cannot be absorbed. So it is important to meet if not exceed the RDA (Recommended Daily Allowances) recommendations for both in order to maintain and improve bone health, and even prevent joint diseases.

Table 6 summarizes the average daily amount
of each needed to prevent disease.[3]

Life Stages Group	Vitamin D (RDA ʋg/day)	Calcium (RDA mg/day)
Infants 0–6 mos.	10	200
7–12 mos.	10	260
Children 1–3 yrs.	15	700
4–8 yrs.	15	1,000
Males 9–13 yrs.	15	1,300
14–18 yrs.	15	1,300
19–30 yrs.	15	1,000
31–50 yrs.	15	1,000
51–70 yrs.	15	1,000
>70y	20	1,200
Females 9–13 yrs.	15	1,300
14–18 yrs.	15	1,300
19–30 yrs.	15	1,000
31–50 yrs.	15	1,000
51–70 yrs.	15	1,200
>70 yrs.	20	1,200
Pregnancy 14–18 yrs.	15	1,300
19–30 yrs.	15	1,000
31–50 yrs.	15	1,000
Lactation 14–18 yrs.	15	1,300
19–30 yrs.	15	1,000
31–50 yrs.	15	1,000

Table 6: Vitamin D and calcium requirements needed
to prevent disease. Adapted from *Nutritional Sciences*,
by Michelle McGuire and Kathy Beerman.

Another recommendation is based on the optimum daily intake (ODI), or what is required not just for disease prevention but also for *optimal* general health. This states that for an adult male or female, these are the daily requirements:[146]

Vitamin D: 1,000 IU
Calcium: 1,000–1,500 mg

For treatment of disease, those dosages are more:[146]

Vitamin D: 2,000 IU
Calcium: 2,000 mg

It's best to get these in natural form. For vitamin D, one would have to increase full solar spectrum sun exposure to a large portion of the skin (think: tank top and shorts) without sunblock, which is called *heliotherapy.* The amount of sun exposure needed is moderate and less than the time required to produce sunburn. [126] There is no finite answer on the exact amount of time needed because it depends on your skin tone, your age, time of day, and where you live. A general rule of thumb is that the darker your skin color, the longer time you need in midday sun versus fair-skinned people may only need three to eight minutes to produce 400 IU. [149] So one would need to be exposed to sun at least two to three times at that rate to result in 1,200 IU vitamin D. If you are unable to meet those requirements either due to lifestyle or injury or illness, then it may be necessary to supplement with vitamin D3 (cholecalciferol), as other forms are less bioavailable for absorption. Of course, eat foods high in vitamin D like fish oils and fatty saltwater fish, such as sea bass, halibut, swordfish, herring, tuna, cod, and sable, in addition to dairy products, if you are tolerant to them. Even sardines, which have not only vitamin D but also calcium, because of eating the bones, can be used to supplement.

I logged a sample day of meals into a nutrition program to assess the nutrient summary where I incorporated dairy, fish, and even organ meat to see if I met the adequate dosages of vitamin D and calcium based on the RDA. Unfortunately, the day of meals did not meet the minimum requirements for either vitamin D or calcium, *not even close.*

There was no section for me to enter sun exposure to assess vitamin D, but at least from a nutrition component, I didn't meet the requirements. What does this mean?

For me it means that if you have a personal history or family history of any joint diseases, cardiovascular disease or osteoporosis, then you should most definitely speak to your health care provider about possible supplementation of Vitamin D3 and calcium in addition to getting full-spectrum sun exposure without sunblock regularly.

Your movement *must* include movement outside with direct exposure to sunrays as often as possible. If you cannot move outside due to weather, job, or injury, then speak to a health care provider about supplementation of vitamin D3 and adjusting your movement as needed.

Remove. Replace. Restore.

Remove heavily refined and processed foods. They are nutrient-depleting, and apparently vitamin D and calcium is hard to come by in food. Remove fear of the sun.

Replace with nutrient-rich whole foods, especially saltwater fish and even bone broth (mentioned in the "Healing" section, recipe in back). Supplement, should your medical or family histories require it as a preventative strategy. Spend time outside in the sunshine in a bathing suit. Don't burn, but expose the cholesterol under your skin to the sunrays to make vitamin D. Healthy exercise is also critical to bone and joint health, even without adequate vitamin D and calcium.

Restore bone health and even improve joint health too.

Soaring Tips

It is true that the best exercise is the one that you will do. All movement counts as exercise, and that must not be forgotten or shamed. Finding the perfect or best exercise for you may take time, trial and error, and patience. No matter what program or routine or athletic competition you choose, it must include getting sun exposure without burning, and also maintaining the range of motion of all your joints (head to your toes).

If you get stuck or injured, a qualified health care provider can help you get back on track. But even through injury, you must always find creative ways to move your body. Movement is life, even during recovery or illness.

Remove. Replace. Restore.

Remove stagnancy.

Replace movements and exercise. Include outdoors in the sunshine regularly.

Restore health.

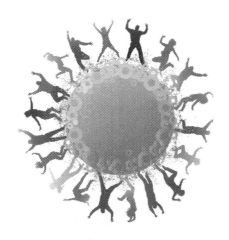

CHAPTER 4: SLEEP WELL

It is a common experience that a problem difficult at night is resolved in the morning after the committee of sleep has worked on it.

—John Steinbeck

Rest and Recovery

I remember in college when my husband and I were dating, after basketball practice and dinner at the dining commons, we would ride our bikes to the library to study. He was a premed double major in history and human physiology, and I was majoring in bioengineering. We would often start strong in our studying, and then we'd literally take a nap—at the table. At the time, I thought it was weird. Now it makes more sense. As we were challenging our brains with different problems, not to mention after a hard practice and high-glycemic food, we would just need some recovery time. After a nap lasting less than thirty minutes usually, we would feel rejuvenated, restored, and ready for more studying until closing time. As I mentioned before, we have been boring for a long time.

Understanding the cycle of sleep may help understand why the nap seemed to help restore and rejuvenate even during those late library hours. The National Sleep Foundation (sleepfoundation.org) describes the following pattern for sleep. The sleep architecture, or makeup, follows a pattern of alternating REM (rapid eye movement) and NREM (non-rapid eye movement) throughout the night in a cycle that repeats about every ninety minutes. Each stage has a unique role.

NREM occurs for approximately 75% of the night and is composed of four stages. Stage one is just between being awake and falling asleep, during which you are in a light sleep. Stage two is the true onset of sleep where you become disengaged from the surroundings and your breathing and heart rate become regular. Your body temperature drops, and so sleep is often easier in a cooler room. (My husband likes this fact because it means he can keep the heater down low so as not to waste money.) Stages three and four are the most restorative sleep stages, where the blood pressure drops, breathing slows further, and muscles relax. The blood flow to the muscles increases, tissue growth and repair begins, and energy is restored. Hormones like growth hormone are released that play a vital role in growth and development.

The second stage of sleep is REM and occurs for only 25% of the night, and first occurs about ninety minutes in to falling asleep. This may occur at longer intervals later into the night. REM sleep provides energy to the brain and body and supports waking performance. During this stage, brain activity increases in the form of dreams, eyes move, and the body becomes immobile and relaxed as the muscles are entirely turned off.

Hormones like cortisol tend to dip around bedtime and increase through the night to stimulate wakefulness in the morning. Sleep is restorative to the immune system and can regulate appetite centers in relation to hormones ghrelin and leptin. We spend nearly a third of our lives sleeping, but it is not unproductive.

Returning to the library again, would our little siesta be restorative? In the short-term, I would say yes. We were getting rapidly into stage three to stage four of sleeping. Although we didn't spend much time sleeping, we were able to feel rested enough to finish our studying. However, during basketball season, I was sure to commit to the truly restorative sleeping that required uninterrupted sleep for hours in order for REM to occur.

As you can see, it is critical to the whole body to turn your consciousness off in order for the reparative process to take place, not to mention that during those REM cycles, I was likely solving some of those engineering problems. Has it ever occurred to you that you struggle with a work or life problem, and after a good night's sleep, you wake up and somehow have a solution in mind? That is the power of good sleep.

Remove. Replace. Restore.
Remove lack of sleep.
Replace with restorative sleep.
Restore the hormonal regulation of sleep. Restore health and even the ability to solve problems.

What Is Enough?

> Rest comes not from the quantity but from the quality of sleep.
>
> —George Gurdjieff

As with anything, the answer to what is enough sleep is complicated, but we will try to simplify it. The answer is "enough is enough." It is impossible to say an exact number for any particular person. The absolute number is dependent on your body, lifestyle, activity level, environment, and goals. As a general guideline, you should sleep when you are tired and wake up naturally to the morning sun. Today, we are staying up later and later, working on computers, cleaning the house, talking on the phone, all when it is dark outside and our homes are lit up with artificial light. Then, once we finally get to bed, we are exhausted but toss and turn, only to have our alarms wake us up before the sun is up.

A rigorous scientific update was performed in 2015 to the National Sleep Foundation's sleep duration recommendations. Table 7 summarizes their results.[150]

Age	Recommended, hrs.	May be appropriate, hrs.	Not recommended, hrs.
Newborns 0–3 mos.	14–17	11–13 18–19	Less than 11 More than 19
Infants 4–11 mos.	12–15	10–11 16–18	Less than 10 More than 18
Toddlers 1–2 yrs.	11–14	9–10 15–16	Less than 9 More than 16
Preschoolers 3–5 yrs.	10–13	8–9 14	Less than 8 More than 14
School-aged children 6–13 yrs.	9–11	7–8 12	Less than 7 More than 12
Teenagers 14–17 yrs.	8–10	7 11	Less than 7 More than 11
Young adults 18–25 yrs.	7–9	6 10–11	Less than 6 More than 11
Adults 26–64 yrs.	7–9	6 10	Less than 6 More than 10
Older adults >65 yrs.	7–8	5–6 9	Less than 5 More than 9

Table 7: Summary of adequate hours of sleep across different age groups per the National Sleep Foundation.

This further demonstrates the point that there is no one single answer that works across the board. It will vary depending on your age, lifestyle, and physiological needs. What I find most fascinating about this data is the fact that my mother has survived thirty years on less than six hours of sleep/ night and is still alive to talk about it. And, as any parent knows, having a young baby is very disruptive of sleep, yet how are all parents not dead from lack of sleep? Our ancestry indicates that we somehow evolved to be a bit flexible throughout our lifetimes, as can be seen by the varying hour requirements of sleep depending on age. The KISS principle of sleeping well allows you to determine for yourself what the magic number is. Depending on the stage of your life, work on making up when you can for the times when you have to lose sleep. For me, it has taken about two years to make up my lost time raising three young children, but I now fall asleep regularly and easily and wake rested, without an alarm, as do all three of my children.

Remove. Replace. Restore.

Remove the habit of pushing past natural sleepiness.

Replace with going to sleep when you are tired and waking up naturally.

Restore your body's natural repair process.

How to Disrupt Sleep Quality

Fatigue is the best pillow.

—Benjamin Franklin

Disrupting sleep is very easy to do. Yet again, in staying true to the KISS principles, you will notice that all things that disrupt sleep quality are often complicated. The quality of your sleep cycle is tightly regulated by a hormonal/endocrine system called the circadian ("around the day") rhythm. [151] Much like the actual sleep cycle, the circadian rhythm is a repetitive process that occurs regularly every twenty hours.

As we discussed earlier, cortisol is one major regulator of sleep, and its peak concentration in the blood is at first rising in the morning. Then it slowly falls throughout the day so that it is at its lowest in the evening before bedtime. These hormones are also tightly regulated by the natural day/light cycle of the sun. Things that may disrupt that cycle are:

- night shift/variable work schedule;[151]
- computer/television screens;[152]
- high-carbohydrate diets;[153]
- caffeine or use of stimulants; and
- alcohol.

If you look closely, all of these factors directly or indirectly affect the cortisol hormone. Shift work and variable work schedules disrupt the cortisol pattern by exposing one's body to light when it should be dark, disrupting that cyclical pattern and expecting sleep when the cortisol levels are the highest during the daytime. Computer and television screens mimic looking into the sun for your retina. So when watching late-night TV, when it should be dark and your cortisol levels are supposed to be the lowest to facilitate sleep, you are actually stimulating wakefulness. High-carbohydrate diets, including alcohol, are a high glycemic load and, therefore, indirectly disrupt the cortisol cycle by stressing the body with insulin production. Even use of stimulants like caffeine can affect the circadian rhythm. You must ask yourself what you need the stimulants for in the first place, and maybe address those issues instead of consuming caffeine. At least, keep consumption of caffeine to a minimum and before noon to allow it to clear your system prior to bedtime. Consuming coffee straight black or with a healthy fat is better than the sugary coffee drinks out there. For me, I find that caffeine use in the morning actually causes me to get extremely tired midafternoon.

It had been thought that exercise later in the day and evening would disrupt sleep, but that does not seem to hold true. [154] So if the evening is the only time for you to exercise or move, then do not worry about it disrupting your sleep. You have far greater improvements in health by exercising than not exercising, so long as you don't miss bedtime.

Many of these factors can be improved, as we will discuss in the next section. However, should your livelihood rely on shift work or variable work schedules, then working closely with a qualified health care provider to work on shifting your circadian rhythm and supplementation would be extremely helpful. At best, manage the things that are in your power to optimize your sleep with the next section.

Remove. Replace. Restore.

Remove sleep-quality disruptors like screen time and high-carbohydrate diets.

Replace with whole-nutrient-rich produce and meats, low lights in the evenings, and regular bedtime. Consult a qualified health care provider if you do shift work to optimize sleep recovery.

Restore reparative sleep and the normal circadian rhythm.

How to Improve Sleep

Sleep is the best meditation.

—Dalai Lama

The absolute first step to improving sleep is to address the first two KISS principles. You must eat well and move well (including being outside in the sunshine) in order to set yourself up for quality sleep. The next steps are simple solutions to modern-day problems.

Keep your bedroom cool. As you progress in the sleep stages, the cooler the temperature, the more likely you are to stay asleep. Keep the ambient temperature between 60–72°F.

Keep your room dark. Blackout curtains are great and necessary, should your job require shift work. Put your alarm clock in the drawer and refrain from bringing your phone into the bedroom. If you can, keep a window blind open that isn't right in your eye to allow morning rays to come in to stimulate you to awaken.

Turn off *all* screens two hours before bedtime. Read a book instead. But if you must use the computer, install an app that dims the computer screen appropriately in tune with the normal cycle of the sun (like the f.lux app). That way, at 9:00 p.m., you aren't looking directly at the sun.

Keep all screens out of the bedroom. Your bed is for sleeping and sex and maybe reading a *real* book by a soft, natural light occasionally.

Get natural sunshine during the day. The full-spectrum sunrays on your skin will help with cholesterol converting to vitamin D, which is also important for improving sleep, in addition to strong bones and joints.

Make it routine. Many sleep books for infants talk about developing a routine in the evenings to get children in the habit of sleeping and being able to fall asleep on their own. The same goes for adults. Think about a plan, then carry it through for a while, and see how you feel. Start with picking a time that works most consistently for you, and then work on the other details.

Eat well. See chapter 2.

Move well. See chapter 3.

Remove. Replace. Restore.

Remove screens from the bedroom and two hours before bedtime.

Replace with regular bedtime. Get regular sunshine. Keep your room dark and cool. Eat well. Move well.

Restore a normal circadian rhythm and restorative sleep.

Soaring Tips

Sleep is beautiful and equally important as the other principles. As with anything, you should make a habit of getting good sleep so that, when sleep is disrupted, you know how to get back on track. My husband, an orthopedic sports and trauma surgeon, often takes call requiring answering phone calls from the hospital for urgent patients through the night. On busy nights, he makes his next day lighter so he can catch up on sleep, and he even goes to bed early the next night. As a family, we try to allow him to sleep whenever he needs. Many jobs require flexibility in sleep, especially for those who work in emergency services (firefighters, nurses, police officers, etc.). Paying attention to the details of the rest of the principles is important because it will help in the times when sleep is disrupted. Periodic sleep disturbance is, in fact, an evolutionary concept, otherwise all parents would be dead after the first week with a newborn.

Remove. Replace. Restore.

Remove sleep disruptors that are in your control.

Replace with regular bedtime in a cool, dark room without screens. Go to sleep when you are tired and wake up naturally. Eat well. Move well. Both will help you to sleep well.

Restore health. Sometimes it isn't perfect, and that's ok. Just get back into the habit, and your body will repair and restore itself while you sleep.

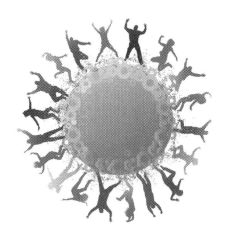

CHAPTER 5: SOAR ON

In life, it's human to fall down; the magic happens when we get back up.

—Grant Korgan, founder of Choose Positivity Now

Purpose and Connection

This KISS principle is probably my most open-ended and flexible. In order to soar in life, you must have *connections* to people in your life and a *purpose* that drives you. For me, my connections are to my husband, my children, my patients, and even my community. I've only recently discovered my purpose to help others gain health and wellness, even through illness and injury. You really must discover what your own purpose and connection is. There is *no* scientific data set that can measure what this is or should be and what it means to you.

Often, discovering what makes you soar requires effort, self-exploration, connecting with new people, trial and error, and often an adverse life event. You don't have to have tragedy to find purpose and connection, but if you don't look for it, you will *never* find it. If you are lucky, your job may be, in part, how you find purpose and connection, but it doesn't have to be that either. Most of the people in my life who I see soaring have, in fact, found a way to find purpose and connection in the job they do.

Let me share a few stories that demonstrate how trying to avoid connection with people leads to unrest and another about tragedy resulting in finding one's purpose.

Raising three young children using these four KISS principles has revolutionized my parenting. At the beginning of our health journey, we made dramatic changes. At that point, I began to realize that although this all made sense and was supported by research (for years and years and years it has been supported), the world wasn't changing as rapidly as our family's transition was. At the time of writing this book, the paleo diet is still considered a fad, despite it actually being a movement of health-seeking behavior. My children's school still offers processed high-carbohydrate foods for snack and lunch. Gatorade and Ring Pops are sold at the Little League snack bars along with Slushees. In school, they still teach the food pyramid in the form of a plate despite all the research to the contrary. There is still a lack of movement tolerated in the classroom, not to mention the loss of daily PE despite the WHO recommendations of one hundred and fifty minutes of moderate to rigorous activity during the week. The middle school students start school at the ungodly hour of 7:00 a.m. requiring 6:00 a.m. bus rides to school. This is a terrible disruption of the circadian rhythm.

At one point, I considered, for like a nanosecond, that maybe I should homeschool my children. That isn't my personality, to be honest, but more importantly, we would have lost the connection with all the kid's friends, the other families, and even the wonderful teachers who truly have gifts that I do *not* have.

A friend of mine, Leah, a mother of four, shared a story about a friend who homeschooled her four children. Leah's friend chose homeschooling for reasons similar to those I indicated. Over time, she began participating in group activities that included other homeschooled children. In an effort to avoid the stress of being a part of public school system (working with others, dealing with conflicting information, and the chaos), she formed a homeschool network through Facebook. What I find most interesting here is the fact that she was trying to avoid all the chaos and conflict of public school, yet the reality was that even removing herself from the public arena, she still felt driven to broaden her connections to more *people.* This is not a statement about whether I agree with homeschooling or whether public school is adequate; it is simply stating that connection to people is critical to being able to soar. Even the most introverted individual has to have people in his or her life, trust me, as a self-discovered introvert who loves many people, just in small doses. This same friend, Leah, has seen me need a nap at a large conference with hundreds of people, yet I learned there and enjoyed myself tremendously.

Now, let's look at a story of purpose. Grant Korgan is a local Reno, Nevada, inspiration. He suffered a tragic spinal cord injury in 2010 while snowmobiling in the backcountry. He has written a book, *Two Feet Back*, that details his life around the injury. Grant found his life's purpose, to inspire others to believe in the power of positivity, in the face of this tragedy. He and his wife, Shawna Korgan, travel the world to inspire others. You can find more about their inspirational story at choosepositivitynow.com. It is an amazing thing to experience, when someone has discovered his or her purpose. Whether or not he needed the tragedy to discover his purpose, we will never know. I certainly hope not. But for him, it was the spark.

For each of us, the spark to discover our purpose may take time, an event, a tragedy, or simply luck. Finding purpose is what matters most. For me, finding my purpose didn't start until that fateful day my father said, "You are morbidly obese and overweight. You need to lose weight, and maybe that will help your sinus problem." However, when I look back at my life from this point, I realize that my purpose has actually been present no matter what stage I was in. One thing that has held constant is the desire to help people, directly. In part, that is why I left bioengineering to go to school to become a physical therapist. I wanted a direct connection to help people. Lab work and computer work did *not* fill my soul. I am one of the lucky ones I guess, because I didn't have a life tragedy, but I don't believe that makes it less meaningful. I am just glad I finally *realized* my purpose.

It took me a while, however. I tried joining different groups. I read self-help books. I even considered joining a church. Yes, I believe in God. I just don't know that joining a church was what I needed to define me as a believer or not. Nor did I feel that it was necessary to live my purpose.

I am drawn to helping people in need, and so is my husband. We enjoy helping people. There have been a few incidents where helping purely means being present when no one else is. A dear family friend, Bonnie, had a health scare that required a hospital stay. Both my husband and I came by to visit while she was in the hospital. Afterward, when she was well recovered, she was profusely grateful for our visits. Our few visits were the highlight of an otherwise stressful situation.

Another time was when our friend Jared was urgently admitted to the hospital for brain surgery. He had been battling headaches for a few weeks, when they suddenly got worse and landed him in the ER. Fortunately, they found the source, and they were able to operate quickly; unfortunately, it was a brain tumor. My husband and I visited him and his wife in the hospital. There wasn't much we could help with, but we knew this was a challenging time for them and simply showed up in support. Despite all the family and many friends they had in town, apparently we were the only ones outside of immediate family who showed up.

Kelly McGonigal said in her book *The Upside of Stress*, "Let yourself be touched by their experience, but also awed by their resilience." Both of us were touched by their experiences, and we continue to be awed by their resilience. Dr. McGonigal describes this as "vicarious resilience" and "vicarious growth." In order for that to occur, the most important factor is genuine empathy. Genuine empathy is the critical factor necessary to have vicarious resilience or growth, feeling not pity but a willingness to experience that person's distress and imagine yourself in their circumstance. In this particular instance, both my husband and I felt empathy with our friend's suffering, not pity. Pity often seems to be an easy way to set up a barrier to someone else's distress and blocks the potential for growth and gaining from his or her strength. To pity someone who is suffering is also to rob that person of his or her growth too. It certainly sounds simple, even if it isn't easy to do.

My husband has naturally always been good at this, especially during and after his medical school training. I never truly appreciated this until I got so wrapped up in my own struggles that I tried to stop him from pursuing his purpose. The experience with our dear friend with the brain tumor further helped me appreciate not only my husband's gift, but also my own.

For my children, I hope that they discover their purpose sooner than I did. It makes life so much more meaningful. More than anything, sooner or later, I just hope that they discover their purpose. Finding my own purpose has allowed me to connect with even more people in even more meaningful ways. Once I discovered my purpose, I was able to remove the fear of failure and replace it with a willingness to try something new, like starting my own practice and starting to write.

There is no recipe for how to soar on in your own life, but it will require purpose and connection. Never fear, though. If all you do is keep connecting to life, the earth, and people, you will be closer to finding purpose.

Remove. Replace. Restore.
Remove fear of failure.
Replace with willingness to try something new. Make a new friend. Join a new club. Try out a new church. Connect to nature, the earth. Join a nonprofit organization. Help another in need, a friend or even a stranger.
Restore life and soar.

Variability

If you want sweet dreams, you've got to live a sweet life.

—Barbara Kingsolver

The beauty of this principle to soar on is the ability for it to vary. Depending on the stage of your life, you may find a different purpose based on where you live, how old you are, what your job is, or something else. You may find that at some point in your life, believing in something bigger than yourself provides solace, and maybe church is the place to be. You may find yourself living in a community that needs help delivering bikes to underprivileged youth. You may find that creating art provides you a release and brings beauty into a world that can never have enough beauty. It may be creating something that solves a problem for someone who can't get into his or her home because of an injury.

Simply find what drives you and makes you happy. It isn't easy to find one's purpose, and you will likely have self-doubt along the way. Let your heart lead, not monetary or social status, and everything will be all right.

Sometimes at different stages of our lives, different gifts will flow through us. I've noticed that ignoring these waves in our lives tends to lead to dissatisfaction. So don't hold back. I have tried to limit the creativity of my middle son at times in order to avoid the chaos in the house. He is prolifically creative and artistic, and it would be detrimental to his development for me to hamper that growth, because I believe it is his purpose. My oldest son's purpose at this stage is to keep the order. I quite enjoy order myself, and I appreciate his help. My daughter's purpose seems to be reminding me how much she loves me. I forget sometimes that I am worth loving the way she loves me.

Remove. Replace. Restore.

Remove the need for things to stay the same.

Replace with flexibility and openness to a new purpose based on where you are in your life at this moment.

Restore happiness and soar.

Soaring Tips

We all have different assets and liabilities to our personalities. Identifying both will help you grow and help you find your purpose and connection. For me, I struggle with name recall. It truly is a handicap of mine. My fear of not remembering someone's name has often stalled my ability to connect with people in my community and in my life. I can't say that I am truly better, but I have adapted, and I acknowledge this fault in order to feel comfortable going to gatherings.

First, I have discussed with my husband a means to help me in conversations, as he remembers almost everything. Second, I can usually recognize faces and remember other details, but out of context, I struggle. I use Facebook to help me link that person to my life, and now I have access to his or her name. Third, I openly admit to people that I have a problem and ask for their names. I find mostly that people sympathize because they have a similar problem, or at least they say so to make me feel better. Either way, it's fine with me. To be totally honest, though I am still embarrassed by this fault, I try not to let it get in the way of me living out the purpose of my life and connecting to people. I hope, whatever your liabilities are, that you don't let it get in the way of living out your purpose either.

Remove. Replace. Restore.

Remove fear.

Replace with acknowledgement of your weakness and a plan.

Restore living your purpose and connecting to people in your community.

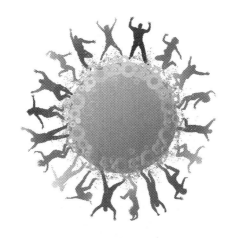

CHAPTER 6: HOW TO PUT THE PRINCIPLES TOGETHER

If you don't start somewhere, you're gonna go nowhere.

—Bob Marley

Start Somewhere

I have laid out four KISS principles to health and wellness. At no point have I said any of these was easy to do. The point really is to provide a framework of reference in order for you to make decisions in your life, simple as that. Should you find yourself stuck and not feeling your best, but you don't know why, then simply start somewhere. For me, my start was actually movement, and then that flowed into eating, then sleeping, and then soaring. It doesn't have to go in that order. But all components are important.

At one point, I would have said that eating well was the most important. I felt that way because you can't move well without adequate energy from nutrients from food, and certainly, your sleep is disrupted if you aren't moving and eating well. Really, the point is that they are all interwoven. So, no matter what you start with, start somewhere. You could choose to focus on sleep because you feel tired all the time, and that would be a good start. But if it doesn't solve the problem, then look next into one of the other KISS principles. And keep moving and adjusting through the KISS principles until you find balance.

If you find yourself stuck, then you may need to seek professional help. One of the reasons I love health care is that to do it right and to do it well you need to address all of these principles. No body system operates in isolation. Traditional health care may have forgotten those words of wisdom, but it is coming back. So if you have a painful condition that limits your movement, seek help from a qualified health care provider, like a physical therapist, who can help with movement. If you have pain, maybe acupuncture, functional medicine, or naturopathy can help give you natural relief, even checking with a medical doctor to help rule out anything scary.

Remove. Replace. Restore.
Remove helplessness.
Replace with one of the KISS principles. Start somewhere. Seek help if you need it so you can keep rolling.
Restore health, wellness, and life.

Wheel

The wheel is come full circle.

—William Shakespeare

My friend, Danielle Litoff, PT, once described all these lifestyle factors with the image of a wheel. Initially, the lifestyle factors were eight in number. Until I realized that the number eight was simply too much for my patients and me to really grasp and remember. When I simplified it to the four KISS principles, things seemed to come together. There are many other visualizations of lifestyle factors out there that include nine, ten, twelve, or more as you break each segment down. They aren't wrong; in fact, they are all correct. It is just that my feeble mind could not remember all of it when I was getting ready to talk with my patients about how to apply them to their lives. Maybe it is all related to my name-recall problem. Either way, it fits my lifestyle to simplify it.

So if we take the four principles and put them together in a wheel, it looks like this:

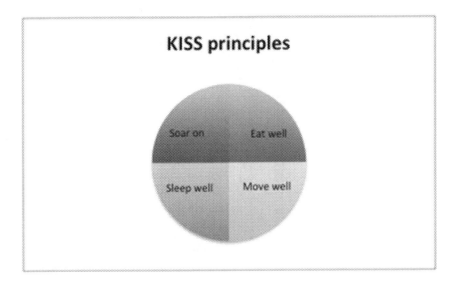

When you have all four principles engaged in your life, the wheel runs smoothly along. What happens when something gets disrupted?

For example, say you need surgery to repair your ligament that was injured from skiing. That will disrupt the "Move Well" section. That doesn't mean your wheel stops rolling altogether, unless you let it. Instead of each principle taking on equal parts, you might set a plan in motion that would increase your connections from soar so your friends and family can help with things you are unable to do. Continue eating well, incorporating more of the nutritional components that facilitate soft tissue healing, like healthy fat, protein, and even homemade bone broth. And, of course, you keep sleeping, sticking to routine and screen-time limits.

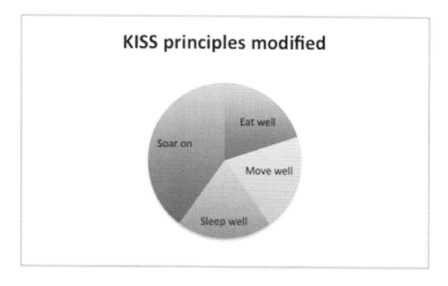

You don't ever stop moving. Maybe you just don't move as much. You still need to move whatever you can and often. Don't forget any one principle altogether, or you will simply stop rolling like a flat tire.

Remove. Replace. Restore.
Remove helplessness.
Replace with other KISS principles temporarily while you get back into balance.
Restore health.

Mishaps

> The wheel that squeaks the loudest is the one that gets the grease.
>
> —Josh Billings

Early in my journey to health, I felt invincible. We had just sold our house, and we were getting ready to move. During that time, I continued working, moving, unpacking, and taking care of kids. I made a few mistakes during that time that ended me in the emergency room with pneumonia when my wheel stopped rolling.

My first mistake was I gave up on sleeping well. I would stay up extra late after the kids were in bed in order to do some unpacking. I did it for weeks in a row, because I did it before we moved and after we moved. I was trying to get it done quickly. Stephen Covey says one of the habits of highly successful people is "fast is slow, and slow is fast." When you try to do things too quickly, you end up with more problems than when you started. Whereas if you take your time to understand and communicate, although it takes longer, you end up successful. In my rush to get it done quickly, I lost sleep and started a steady decline into a bigger problem.

The second mistake I made was I stopped eating well. I would make the kids dinner, but I didn't take the time to sit and eat myself. Instead, I used Dr Pepper as my meal replacement. Not a good choice, and I knew it, but I truly thought that since I was so "healthy" that my body could handle it temporarily.

The third mistake I made was I didn't call on my connections for help. I tried to do it all by myself, being the fierce independent women that I am. I simply couldn't do it all alone while my husband took trauma call and was gone covering all the athletic teams he was committed to taking care of.

About the only thing I did right was moving well. You get plenty of exercise moving boxes and unpacking, but it may not be considered healthy, given the state of everything else. I was, in fact, lucky I didn't injure myself.

So one night, I went to bed, and suddenly my left shoulder was hurting when I was lying down. It seemed really weird. I took a deep breath, and it hurt worse. I told my husband, and we didn't know what that was about, except it was only 7:30 p.m. and I was already sleeping. We thought all I needed was rest since I had been stressed with the move. I was beginning to slow down. I noticed that I was more and more tired right after dinner. I had a cold that I couldn't quite kick, and I even started to get fevers around 7:00 or 8:00 p.m. at night. I got so fatigued at one point that I called in sick to work, because all I had energy to do was get the kids to school and go back home to bed.

The next night, I was on the couch watching TV after putting the kids to bed. My husband was on call and not home. As I was sitting there, I got a pain in my ribcage. It was so severe it brought tears to my eyes. My fever had come back, and every time I took a breath, the pain got worse. Now I was scared. I called my friend who was in medical school at the time and talked to her about it since I didn't want to disturb my husband working. She told me that I needed to get checked out. It wasn't normal for a "healthy" person to continue with fevers and now this pain.

We ended up in the ER, and they ran tests and took pictures of my lungs. They said I had the flu. I just needed to rest. I think I'd fooled even my husband, because I was working so hard to keep it all together that I didn't really look that sick. Then, when they were ready to discharge me, that lung pain came back, and the doctor looked at me and said, "You don't look good. Are you feeling ok?" I said no. I felt terrible. They listened to my lungs again, and it was as if I was just progressing into full pneumonia in front of them. They heard crackles in my lungs when I breathed this time.

In medical school and even physical therapy school, you practice listening to lungs. I had never truly heard crackles until that day. It had been years since my husband had heard them, but he could too. They still discharged me, but this time with broad-spectrum antibiotics.

I slowly recovered, but it took a long time and a huge effort to get back on track again. Living the KISS principles truly helped me. I did need supplementation to get the healthy bugs back in my gut and special supplements to heal my leaky gut. I got extra sleep, and I kept moving without overexerting myself until I settled back into a healthy state.

Remove. Replace. Restore.

Remove rushing to get it all done in a short time and ignoring your body's signals.

Replace with patience, a steady pace, and touching on all the principles habitually.

Restore health and efficiency.

Soaring Tips

The KISS principles are simple, but they are easy to ignore. When you ignore them, things start to break down. It may not happen overnight, but if you make a habit of ignoring the principles, you will falter. It may not be pneumonia, but you are lucky if you can catch your falter soon enough. Always make it a habit to try and touch on each principle *every day*, and you will save yourself from falls like this. Yet, if you do, these principles will help you to get rolling again.

Remove. Replace. Restore.
Remove the idea that you are a superhuman.
Replace with KISS principles daily. Make them a habit.
Restore health and prevent disease.

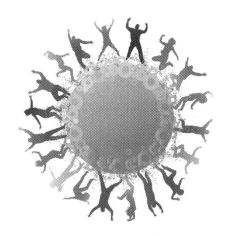

CHAPTER 7: WHAT ABOUT STRESS?

How you think about something can transform its effect on you.

—Kelly McGonigal, PhD, *The Upside of Stress*

Fact of Life

My health journey truly started in 2012 and continues today and always. As I was able to dial in my nutritional habits to truly "Eat Well," exercised regularly with CrossFit and simple movements to "Move Well," I focused on getting adequate rest consistently to "Sleep Well" and was always working on how to "Soar On" by connecting with friends or family, reading, writing, or a combination. The one area where I struggled was "Stress Management."

What is stress?

"Stress (noun): 1. a strain or straining force; a) force exerted upon a body, that tends to strain or deform its shape b) the intensity of such force, usually measured in pounds per square inch c) opposing reaction or cohesiveness of a body resisting such force 2. Emphasis; importance; significance 3. a) Mental or physical tension or strain b) urgency, pressure." [1]

So my health guide at this time in my life, Meg Mangano, RD, was offering up strategies to decrease my stress. The first was to cut out my processed sugar, which included chocolate. Yes, I am a closet chocolate eater. When the going gets rough after the kids come home from school, my hand goes into the chocolate bag for a quick dopamine release. This worked all right, but I always fell prey to it during the hours when all kids were home from school and we had homework, sports, dinner, bedtime routine, and whatever else needed to get done. It wasn't a productive strategy, not to mention it put extra pounds on me over time.

The next step was to try meditation to deal with stress. I tried meditating my stress away. I practiced in the morning, evening before bed, and sometimes during the day while the kids were at school. I even tried walking meditation because sitting still for extended periods made me feel antsy and lazy. (I had things to do! Don't forget my pregnancy story.)

I like meditation mostly, but I still felt stressed. Until it dawned on me that being a mother, the role I treasure the most, was what stressed me out. And I couldn't "manage" the stress away because my kids were my kids and I loved them. I was defeated. I was going to suffer from the damage of stress no matter how well I did anything else in my life to be healthy.

I went to our bedroom and cried. I cried serious tears of absolute defeat. My husband came in and found me. How in the world could I admit that the very things I loved were the same things that were killing me? How come all mothers have not died of stress before me? That sounded so crazy. I was doomed. I knew. Objectively it really sounded crazy, because I had a beautiful life. And I fear that if my children read this that they think it means I didn't love them or that I didn't enjoy mothering them. That is so far from the truth! However, the fact is that motherhood is stressful. And life is stressful. It is a fact of life.

Remove. Replace. Restore.
Remove fear of stress.
Replace acceptance of stress as a fact of life.
Restore the ability to live today.

Acceptance

Happiness can exist only in acceptance.

—George Orwell

One day, a physical therapy colleague of mine shared a TED talk with me given by Kelly McGonigal, PhD. A TED is a nonprofit organization devoted to spreading ideas where Technology, Entertainment and Design (TED) converge. In Dr. McGonigal's talk, she discussed her experience with stress as a health psychologist and professor. She shared how too much stress leads essentially to heart disease, stroke, and potentially, death. Scare tactics. If something is going to kill you, won't you try to avoid it? I did the same in my practice and believed it for my own life. In physical therapy, we talk about optimal body mechanics and ergonomics. And if you aren't able to lift properly, your back will give out, and your intervertebral disks will degenerate to nothing. Scare tactics.

Turns out, if you believe something is bad for you, it will be bad for you. "The effect you expect is the effect you get," Kelly McGonigal wrote in *The Upside of Stress*. If you believe something won't work for you, it won't. If you believe you have failed, then you fail. It is similar to the placebo effect. If you believe the white pill is going to cure your disease, it will have positive effects on your illness.

Two articles support these statements related to the effect of mind-set on stress. One was done to test the whether the gut peptide ghrelin (an indicator of satiety or feeling full after eating) would vary depending on the mind-set in which a person consumes a particular food. Ghrelin levels were measured under two conditions of consuming a 380-calorie milkshake under the pretense that it was either a 620- calorie "indulgent" shake or a 140-calorie "sensible" shake. There was a steeper decline in ghrelin after consuming the "indulgent" shake, indicating that the person was satiated. Yet when they consumed the "sensible" shake, the ghrelin levels indicated that the subject was still hungry. [155] The shakes were exactly the same, yet labeled differently. There appears to be a meaningful physiological response to food based on the psychological mind-set. Mind over matter, right?

The same investigator, Crum, also examined the difference of mind-set as it related to exercise. She tested eighty-four female attendants working in seven different hotels for healthy variables affected by exercise. Those who were educated about how their job met all the requirements for an active lifestyle based on the Surgeon General's recommendations were found to have lost weight, lowered blood pressure, and decreased body mass index as compared to those in the control group after only four weeks. [156] Those that had the education about how their jobs *fulfilled* the Surgeon General recommendations versus the control group which only got education *about* the receommendations. The only difference was their *mind-set intervention.*

After that evening when I truly felt my kids were stressing me to death (I jest here. It's ok to laugh.), I realized that stress was everywhere. And it wasn't *all* bad. I changed my *mind-set* about stress. In fact, if we look at all four components of health and wellness that I have laid before you, every single one of them has "stress" as an overlying part. And maybe I was actually addicted to it? (Why else would I try to write a book, work part-time, and start a business while raising three children? It's probably because my brain and my body thrive on stress.)

Remove. Replace. Restore.
Remove scare tactics.
Replace with a new mind-set.
Restore the ability to thrive with stress.

Stress Is Health

The greatest weapon against stress is our ability to choose one thought over another.

—William James

Eating well includes stress. Plants have evolved over years to present different biological chemicals that prevent other organisms, like insects and predators, from eating the plant. Most of these chemicals do not actually kill the organism but stimulate a response in the nervous system to indicate a bad taste. The nervous system via the taste buds of the predator would indicate the potential toxin, a stress response.

As human evolution goes, we evolved to eat a wider range of plants as we became tolerant of those toxins. These toxins, or bitter-tasting fruits and vegetables, activate signaling pathways that, in fact, protect against disease. So the bitterness of, say, a fresh raspberry would be designed to discourage an organism from eating it, yet it is packed with antioxidants, which are antiaging components.

Additionally, raw vegetables and fruits contain bacteria that, again, it would seem to be ill-advised to consume, yet they contribute to our overall health by taking residence in our gut. These bacteria can assist in fighting off infection, help break down food, and even provide additional vitamins for our benefit. So in a manner, the "stress" of eating a raw plant food is, in fact, *healthful*.

Moving well includes stress. When we discuss movement or exercise, we also bring along physical "stress." If you want to gain muscle bulk and strength, you have to lift weights. You start light and progress to heavier weights. The soreness that ensues while you progress is stressful to the muscle fibers, but that actually stimulates a response of the myoblasts (cells that synthesize muscle) to produce more muscle fibers, therefore making the muscle stronger. You can't gain *strength* without progressively stressing the muscle. The same is true for bone strength. You have to load the bone with weight-bearing loads in order to stimulate the osteoblasts (cells that synthesize bone) that respond to mechanical stress and produce more bone.

Sleeping well includes stress. The effort to modify your life in order to improve sleep is a challenge, a stress. Often we have things out of our control that prevent our ability to sleep continuously. When you look at sleep directly, though, your brain is never shut off entirely, nor is your body. Although your consciousness is taking a break, your body continues to repair, remodel, and clean up. It is, in a way, continually stressed as you sleep.

Soaring on includes stress as well. In order to soar, you likely will be required to have some mental strain. Finding one's purpose and connecting with people requires trial and error, give and take, or pressure. Not only that, but also it evolves over time, requiring you to change or find a new hobby or passion, depending on your current life situation. Again, it evolves, and change produces stress and requires change or response.

Remove. Replace. Restore.
Remove fear of stress.
Replace with a healthy relationship with stress. Normal stress helps produce strong bones, muscles. Stress is a component of healthful food. Even during rest, our body is busy being stressed as it repairs.
Restore the ability to soar today.

Interwoven

> I know there is strength in the differences between us. I know there is comfort where we overlap.
>
> —Ani DiFranco

If we look at the four KISS principles and stress as two independent wheels it looks like this:

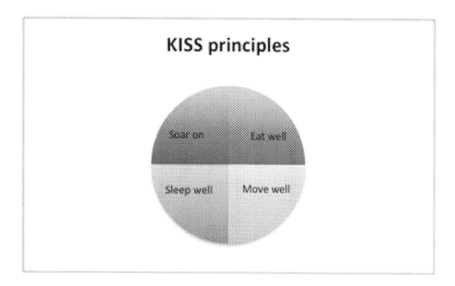

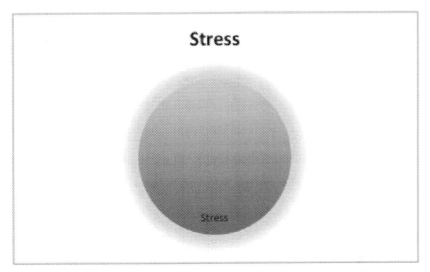

If we overlap them to make them one, it looks more like this:

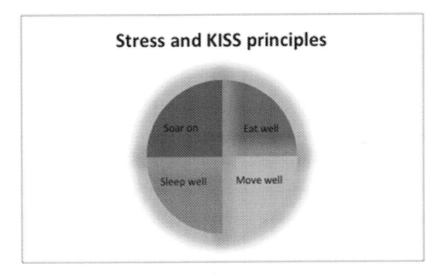

That is one radiant pie chart! It demonstrates my point so well. You can't have life without stress. Stress makes things brighter and more meanigful. My husband even shared this with me. He asked me, "Do you know how to make a diamond? It takes two things." I wasn't quite sure where he was going with this as it related to stress and health, but I said, "Coal and pressure. Oh! Stress!" To make a diamond, you need coal and, yes, stress.

I don't mean to make light of the impact stress has on health altogether, but certainly I think we give it too much credit and allow it to negatively impact our lives. We do need to acknowldege and respond to it using the four KISS principles and give yourself ample time to process stressful life events.

Remove. Replace. Restore.
Remove attempts to avoid all stress.
Replace with image of a diamond.
Restore radiance.

Connection

> Communication—the human connection—is the key to personal and career success.
>
> —Paul J. Meyer

Let's look at a child's response to a stressful event like the loss of a pet. We recently lost one of our dear cats at the young age of two and a half years. This is the first pet my children had truly had a close connection with, and they felt the loss. My oldest son, god bless him, found the deceased cat one morning. He reflexively cried. I have yet to see him cry with such emotion. The stress of the loss and visual of death resulted in crying. He reached out to *connect*. It was instinctual to reach out for a connection with someone he trusted to express his sorrow and anger. And obviously I attempted to provide him with a means for him to share his feelings. But I also was sure to provide one of his favorite meals for dinner, sushi along with a healthy green smoothie. Although he was traumatized, he still spent some time outside, being active and moving, and we went to bed early that night. We hit every one of the four principles that day in hopes of simply supporting him through this stressful time.

As we age, it gets more complicated, or I guess we make it more complicated. One of my urges was to offer up a night out for some frozen yogurt or ice cream. And if I had lost a spouse, I may have been tempted to lean on some alcohol to numb the pain. I can't say either one is wrong or right, because I have both eaten sweets and used alcohol to deal with stress in the past. But it is no secret that neither of those responses would result in anything positive. Both using food and using alcohol are easy and temporary responses. They both are by no means an acknowledgement and honororing of the stressful event.

This may be an oversimplification of stressful life events, but I still believe the fundamentals (the four KISS prinicples) are a great guide to get started with in addressing a stressful situation, no matter the severity. It may require assistance from a licesened professional, but that is still connection (soar).

I would like to acknowledge a few conditions where stress is *harmful* whether or not you have shifted your "mind-set." A few examples would be alcoholism, abusive relationships—physical or mental, traumatic incidents, or physical injury like fractures. All would require professional help. I encourage anyone suffering from these to reach out to a professional for help. These conditions are more common than I may appreciate, but certainly everyday life stress is likely suffered by everyone, and it is this that I speak to.

It makes a difference whether you choose to believe that stress is harmful or stress is enhancing. The fact is, experiencing stress simply means that you are *alive*. You *cannot* manage stress and make it go away. Trust me: I have personally tried. And it nearly killed me. (I jest. I just thought it was killing me.) You must accept that stress is a part of living. Making peace with that simple fact will allow you to use stress to your benefit.

Remove. Replace. Restore.

Remove attempts to dampen stressful life events with food and alcohol.

Replace with acknowledgement. Reach out to a loved one or professional help especially if you find yourself in a "stress is harmful" situation. Support yourself positively using the KISS principles.

Restore the connections in your life to carry you through everyday stress.

Soaring Tips

If you are reading this book, I don't doubt that you have experienced stress in your life or that you feel you have a lot of it currently. But cheers to you for reaching for a book that hopefully helps you use stress to make something happen in your life.

Stress can make you change how you eat, so you feel better. Emotional stress can be relieved with exercise, and mechanical stress can stimulate muscle growth. Stress can push you to reach out to a loved one, a good friend, or someone to *connect* with, soar. Stress brings people together while controlling and demonizing stress tears people apart.

Let me offer up another definition of stress:

Life, connection, strength, and the ability to change and learn

Acknowledge and *honor* the stressful events in your life, and use the four KISS principles to help you find your balance and connection again. What that looks like is different for every one of us.

Remove. Replace. Restore.

Remove fear of stress.

Replace with acknowledgement. Honor stressful life events and consider your response. Stress means you are alive and living. Reach out to a friend, a family member, or a licensed professional. Focus energy on other components of the four KISS principles to help you through stressful life events. Should you find yourself in a "stress is harmful" situation, seek professional help as soon as possible.

Restore a sense of community. Connections to the people around you often will be invaluable in moving through life, but you have to be open to them.

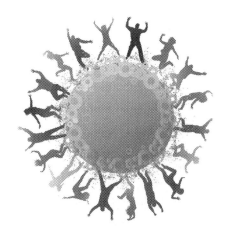

CHAPTER 8: SOARING FINAL THOUGHTS

Because I Said I Would

Because I said I would.

—Alex Sheen

A few years ago, my husband and I were traveling on Southwest Airlines. You know that magazine on the airplane? Well, I have a crazy story. We got some very *useful* and *life-changing* information from that magazine. I know. I can't believe it either.

There was an article about a young man named Alex Sheen who had recently lost his father. Sparked by the loss, he started a nonprofit organization, really a social movement, called *because I said I would*. This movement is dedicated to the betterment of humanity by means of *accountability*. He provides promise cards to those requesting them that say, "because I said I would," as a means of keeping track of what you promise to do. He has a TED talk, and shares his promises and stories of others who have been helped too. I have one of his cards from the same Southwest magazine taped to my computer screen so both my husband and I see it daily (www.becauseisaidiwould.com).

Accountable as an adjective, defined by *Webster's New World Dictionary*, is "1. Obliged to account for one's acts; responsible, 2. Capable of being accounted for; explainable."

Since reading that article, I work conscientiously to follow through with my commitments, being accountable. I do not make statements or commitments verbally or otherwise without attempting to thoroughly think about my ability to carry through with them before agreeing. This means that sometimes I have to say no to things, but really it keeps me accountable. I try not to speak just to fill empty air space, and I work carefully to keep from making empty threats to my children. I am not perfect, but I am certainly more aware of my words since reading this story than I was before.

One summer day, my husband and I attempted to summit Mt. Rose. After making a wrong turn and missing the summit, we said that we would try again, and we would take our kids to the waterfalls. A few weeks later, we completed both, purely "because I (we) said I (we) would." We are practicing the art of "because I said I would" for ourselves, for our family, and hopefully for the further betterment of humanity.

It was work. It was effort. It was worth it. More than anything, we found the joy of being accountable for our word of commitment to each other. Making a promise to yourself and seeing it through is one of the most rewarding feelings. And making a promise to another person and following through is even more rewarding, so long as it isn't for financial gain (think: buying a product versus raising money for a cause).

Local hero Grant Korgan has this down. He circumnavigated the rim of the great Lake Tahoe to raise money for a wonderful cause, the High Fives Foundation (http://highfivesfoundation.org). The High Fives Foundation supports the dreams of mountain-action sports athletes by raising injury prevention awareness while providing resources and inspiration to those who suffer life-altering injuries. *Why?* Because he said he would and, in doing so, makes humanity better.

Parenting accountability is probably the best teacher I have encountered for myself. Let me share a parenting story I experienced during my journey to health. At one point as I tried to decrease the exposure to BPA (a toxic, hormone-like chemical that is leached from plastic wares and bottles) in the household, I purged all of our plastic bottles and containers that were not labeled BPA-free and replaced them with stainless steel or glass. I discussed with the kids why we were doing it. We are religious about carrying water bottles with us. Why? Because it is good for the environment, because it is better for us, and because we said we would avoid plastic.

One day at the baseball field, we had forgotten to bring water bottles. In the heat of the day and the lateness of our arrival, we did not have time to return home to get them. Fortunately, I had cash on me, which is unusual, because I usually use my credit card all the time. I sent my son to the dreaded snack bar to get four bottled waters. They all stopped and stared at me. For a moment I didn't understand, until I realized they were worried about the plastic. Having listened to me, they knew this was a conflict from what I had said earlier. They were holding me accountable for what I told them about plastic and BPA. And they should have. We discussed that in living life in this world, sometimes you have to compromise, and you make a choice. The heat of the day put us at risk for dehydration during the game in the Nevada sun, and the risk of this one-time exposure to BPA in the bottled water, although not ideal, was certainly better than dehydration. For sure, it was the best choice we could make, given our options of soda, Gatorade, or Slushee. In hindsight, I could have chosen an empty cup with a straw for the baseball player, but I didn't think of it at the moment. Hopefully, I will next time. What I learned was that the kids, all three, were keeping me accountable.

My prepaleo wholefoods life was full of confusion for the children. I often see other parents falling into the same patterns. How often did we go out to eat as a family, order the healthiest dinner for the kids, expect them to eat theirs, and then order myself a soda and not allow them to have one? How often did I order myself a salad for dinner and then let the kids eat mac and cheese? It seems impossible now to look back and wonder how I offered such conflictive choices. I certainly can't set a standard for children and not hold myself to it or hold myself to a different standard than my children. Nor can I ask my patients to do something if I can't live by the same principle, even if it looks different.

My initial health journey looked like perfect paleo, where I removed all dairy, all grains, and all legumes. Where I settled nutritionally in our healthy state as a family looks like paleo with some dairy and occasional gluten-free grains, traditionally prepared. Should we choose to stray from that, my children hold me accountable. It sparks a conversation about why we made that choice or how we made the choice. This accountability actually makes me a better person, even with my imperfections.

My goal in writing this book is to share information, insights, and stories that may help you or make you think so you can make informed decisions. And I will continue to work on being accountable for the words I write and say, both here and for my children, for my family, for my patients, and really for the betterment of humanity.

As parents, it is critical that we are accountable for our actions, behaviors, and words. You know the children will remind you of what you said, so don't say it if you don't mean it. As health care providers we must demonstrate the behavior that we are seeking in our patients. As health care authority figures for patients and as parents to our children, we cannot say, "Do as I say, not as I do." That is not an effective strategy.

By being accountable for our words, our actions, our behaviors, we can not only make the world a better place, but also maybe we can even improve the health of our community.

Remove. Replace. Restore.

Remove mindless commitments, fear of commitment, and fear of failure.

Replace with accountability. Think before your speak. Take yourself and others seriously. Be accountable for the benefit of humanity, not personal financial gain.

Restore humanity and even health.

Shame and Guilt

> It is not the critic who counts; not the man who points out how the strong man stumbles, or where the doer of deeds could have done them better. The credit belongs to the man who is actually in the arena, whose face is marred by dust and sweat and blood; who strives valiantly … who at the best knows in the end the triumph of high achievement, and who at the worst, if he fails, at least fails while daring greatly.
>
> —Theodore Roosevelt

As any parent knows, shame and guilt are inevitable. You are trying to do your best as a parent, but then you yell at your child out of frustration. Not only have you accidently shamed your child, but also then, the guilt you feel afterward is terrible. How about all those working parents who miss their children's ballet recitals because the parents were stuck at important meetings? Or when you are trying to live whole foods–inspired, but you just can't make a meal from scratch today, so you grab a gluten-free pizza instead?

To the outsider, all of these incidents could be considered failures. Truly, our worst critics are ourselves. Brene Brown, PhD, in her book *Daring Greatly* discusses the importance of shame. Dr. Brown documents and shares experiences related to the benefits of shame. Much like stress, it is important to acknowledge the shame tendencies in your own life and use them to your benefit. In order to dare greatly one must redefine success, reintegrate vulnerability, and seek support. [157] If we look at a few of the examples listed above, how could the shame be turned around into something positive?

In the case of losing control of your voice by yelling, one could stop and kneel down to their levels and simply apologize and ask for forgiveness. We are human and mistakes happen. My dear friend, Amy, gave me some words of wisdom on my wedding day about what makes for a happy marriage. She said, "Never yell at each other unless the house is on fire." The next wise words were "when you have done something wrong, be ready to admit it and ask for forgiveness." These words not only apply to marriage but also to raising children and really to any relationship. It is important for our children to learn about how to deal with mistakes. We are all human. To ignore the mistake is to take the easy way out and avoid the benefits of shame.

In the case of missing a child's recital, how about simply apologizing for missing it and then asking him or her all about it? Let the child relive it for you as if you were there. And in the case of your buying gluten-free pizza, maybe no apology is really needed except to try and plan a little better for next time. Hop right back on the healthy-food train at the next meal. Maybe even think of the best choices when eating out. Pair the gluten-free pizza with a large salad or healthy vegetables, and your meal is not half bad. The point is life happens. Acknowledge it when it does, and get back on track as soon as you can.

Let me share another experience of my son's. We had a few boys over, playing. At some point, they were playing at the tree house, and my middle son felt as though his older brother was teasing him. He reacted by throwing a rock. It was intended for his brother, but it hit his friend on the cheek. Nobody was physically harmed, but my son came in and said he needed to have the playdate over because he was a horrible person; he was shaming himself, and he felt guilty. Obviously, there needed to be a consequence, and, fortunately, at that moment, I was able to keep my voice level. I sent him to his room to take a few moments to settle down so we could talk about it.

He continued to shame himself, saying he couldn't control himself so he should never have playdates again, that maybe he wouldn't be good at school anymore because he couldn't control himself. We talked about how every situation is a learning experience, how he would learn more about better self-control next time, and how we should use words instead of a physical response first. The playdate for him was over, but he then needed to apologize to his friend and ask for forgiveness. He also then needed to apologize to his friend's mother for the incident. I was really proud of how he handled it, despite his self-shaming. He made himself vulnerable to both his friend and his friend's mother, apologizing and asking for forgiveness. He asked for support because he wasn't sure he could do it alone. I stood beside him. It was hard work, and he understood that his actions potentially hurt many people he cared about. There were tears, hugs, forgiveness, and positive learning experiences in the span of an hour.

Too often, we ignore these opportunities for learning for the easy route of a pity response. If you make a mistake, acknowledge it and try to repair the damage. Controlling it with shame, punishment, or guilt is a quick resolution, but far from ideal. Our definition of success as win or lose when it relates to life and people needs rethinking. Success can be win-win in life, in business, and in health care.

Remove. Replace. Restore.
Remove shame and guilt.
Replace with daring greatly. Acknowledge the shame and guilt. Redefining success for win-win. Be vulnerable. Apologize. Ask for forgiveness. Seek support from others you trust when you need it most.
Restore humanity, learning, and community.

Perfection

Done is better than perfect.

—Sheryl Sandberg, *Lean In: Women,*
Work, and the Will to Lead

Perfection is defined by Merriam-Webster as "a condition of complete excellence, as in skill or quantity, or completely correct or accurate." That word and definition has a lot of pressure. In anything other than a simple math problem of 1 + 1 = 2, I don't see any perfection in life, except to say perfect imperfection. For me, the beauty of many things in life is that, in fact, they aren't perfect.

Certainly there are cases where near perfection may be necessary, like in the operating room, but even then that is an unrealistic expectation. When you break your wrist and the doctor sets it to near perfect, that is great. No matter how good the surgery or setting, it is never as perfect as what you started with, but it's not a problem. My father, the ear, nose, and throat surgeon, sometimes said, "The enemy of good is better." If you put something back together and it looks good, and then you try to make it look perfect, you often undo the good work and actually make it worse.

For example, when you are doing your hair with product, blow-drying, and curling iron, you can't seem to get the one curl to go the right way. As you keep curling and spraying, suddenly all the curl is gone, because you now have too much stuff in it. Fortunately, you could start over with a shower, but you might not have enough time. For many things in life, you don't get a do-over.

I have heard people say that they can't do "perfect paleo like Carolyn." I don't know what that means. There is nothing about my life that is "perfect paleo." Fortunately, I am not truly allergic to soy or peanuts or gluten, but I do keep them to a minimum. If by "perfect" you mean after the soccer game my family and I skip the donut, then yes, I guess we are "perfect." Because we would much rather celebrate a win with a high five and congratulations than a food item. Should we really want to celebrate a birthday or something with a sweet treat, we do! We choose something that won't make us feel bad or guilty or sick, because the point is to *celebrate.*

If you set yourself up for perfection, you set yourself up for failure. If I expected myself to be 100% compliant with eating whole foods and avoiding *all* processed foods, I would be living alone in the brush. I want a lifestyle I can maintain. When I performed the two-week whole foods eating trial that I mentioned in the introduction, people pretty consistently met 80:20 perfection. That meant that they ate whole foods (80%) and had a few cheat meals (20%) of the time. What is more important here is that you *did not* need 100% perfection to see improvement in health, wellness, and even pain levels.

That is pretty cool. Phew. Take a load off. Take the pressure bands off my head. I do not need to be perfect! Thank goodness. Now, I am not promoting that you don't strive to do the best that you can, and making some lifestyle changes is important. I strive to make a majority of my food whole nutrient-rich food. I strive to make exercise and movement a part of my daily life. I strive for quality sleep every evening. How perfect each of those things is, is different every day. I strive to address each principle regularly, to make a habit. I don't strive for perfection. Fortunately, my healthy state at this moment allows it, but some don't have that luxury. Be cautious when allowing "imperfect" to become just continuing old bad habits.

If you suffer from a debilitating disease, you may need to focus on better than good, because your life depends on it, but it likely won't be forever. You will have made some very good habit adjustments along the way that will keep you moving forward. And you will find where your imperfect decisions are ok and when they aren't. For example, in some cases, dairy may trigger the inflammatory response you are trying to avoid, and that is where your body needs better than good enough, but more perfect. Yet maybe a cracker with gluten in it is less inflammatory for you.

My laundry is not always clean, folded, or put away. My food is healthy, but not always perfect. I don't always remember to use stress to my advantage. I forget. I try again the next time. I don't always remember to use shame and guilt to have a positive learning experience, but I try better each time. In part, that is why I wrote this book: to let my children know what I was striving for despite being imperfect and to have something I can reference when I forget. My life is imperfect, but I am glad someone sees it as perfect. Because the fact is that we are all the same, imperfect people in an imperfect world trying to do the best we can.

Remove. Replace. Restore.

Remove perfect expectations of yourself, they are unrealistic.

Replace with realistic lifestyle changes and improved habits. Make the best choices you can because it's the right thing to do, not because it is easy.

Restore happiness and health.

Booby Traps

Fool me once, shame on you. Fool me twice, shame on me.

—Randall Terry

"Booby trap" is defined in Webster's dictionary as "any scheme or device for tricking a person unawares." It is honest enough to not be lying, but dishonest enough to trick you into something you might not otherwise do if you had all the information. I would like you to be aware of a few booby traps that I have identified so you don't have to fall prey to them. Let me explain.

Today I went to the grocery store. I do it a lot. Yes, living the KISS principles does mean I have to grocery shop more than I used to. I have learned over time to keep my eyes averted in certain areas to avoid the grocery booby traps. For example, the entry to the new and remodeled grocery store in town has all kinds of fresh fruits jammed into the doorway. That's ok, I guess. Except I know they do it because they want me, mother of three kids, to buy some healthy fruit so I just may buy some more junk once I get in. Because statistics show that if I (a mother) buy "healthy," I will have checked "healthy" off my list and be more likely to fall for the potato chips later. I am not falling for it, even if I buy the bananas in the entry.

Then in the health food section, I see "Whole Grain," "Organic," "Vitamins," "Omega 3," "Paleo," "No High-Fructose Corn Syrup," or "Gluten-Free." And if you pick up most of these packaged and processed items and actually read the ingredients, they still have tons of ingredients I can't pronounce or understand why they are even included. I want organic ketchup with tomatoes in it. Not with agave or organic cane sugar or vegetable oil or whatever else they try to sneak in there to make it sugar sauce. So *read* the *labels* on everything, even if the front says it's healthy.

When I go to check out, I don't want to see rows of candy bars. Because you know when I am shopping, I am probably hungry, and I probably have a kid or two in tow that will be hungry also. I find this booby trap just cruel and unusual punishment. How many times have you seen (or even been) the poor parent in the checkout line with kids grabbing all the junk? They don't want to make a bigger scene, so they give in. And I don't care if you are a fancy store that carries higher quality "junk food." It is the same problem. In order to deal with this booby trap, maybe the best idea is not to shop hungry. Regular whole foods eating does help regulate the blood sugar so you don't get the highs and lows as often.

It's only slightly better when the healthy bars are on one side and the unhealthy bars on the other. I know Epic bars exist, and if I need them, I will go get them. But if we are honest, when I am headed to the checkout line, I think I imply that I am actually done shopping. Maybe this is why I like to do so much online shopping, to avoid the booby traps.

I find booby traps at sporting events for the kids. Junk food is everywhere. Candy bars, Ring Pops, sodas, Slushees in crazy "flavors" (which, by the way, is just code for chemicals to trick your brain into believing it tastes like strawberry—if you didn't already know, there are no strawberries in your strawberry Slushee from the concession stand). We can't expect our children or even most adults to turn away from this, not to mention the snacks after games. I have already touched on the booby traps at the sporting events. The worst part is, it is other mothers doing the booby-trapping. I appreciate the effort behind wanting to bringing a sweet treat to celebrate the game, such as "sugar tubes" with the name "yogurt," Gatorade, or crackers, all in the name of fun and goodwill. However, I ask, "Why does my toddler need anything but water after T-ball?" Ok, maybe some orange slices, but not really. He just stood around.

There is even a game called BeanBoozled. I have to admit it is fun and a great marketing strategy. There are jelly bean colors that look alike, but taste different. For example, one brown jelly bean tastes like chocolate and another similarly brown-colored jelly bean tastes like canned dog food. Totally gross.

The ingredients are even worse. What a learning experience—to see how the chemicals and marketing can trick our taste buds.

I guess it's not a booby trap anymore if you are no longer unaware. You will find booby traps even in the fitness world too. Not everyone, but many people like to play into our personal vulnerabilities, especially the things we shame and guilt ourselves over—like how we look and what we eat. Having the KISS principles in your pocket anywhere you go will help you sort through these booby traps more easily.

Remove. Replace. Restore.

Remove marketing trickery, brain games, playing to my vulnerabilities.

Replace with awareness. They can only trick us if we let them in. Put your guard up. *Always* look at the ingredients.

Restore health, control, and peace because there will be fewer temper tantrums in the checkout line. Just saying.

Tips for Parents

At the end of the day, the most overwhelming key to a child's success is the positive involvement of parents.

—Jane D. Hull

I transitioned my children from the SAD diet at the young ages of seven, five, and three. From my experience, it primarily took consistency and some explanation on simply eating to feel better and to not be sick. Whether or not I wanted to lead this family to health when I became a mother, it is what I ended up doing and continue to do.

Here are a few things that I helped make the transition more successful for our family:

1. *Consistency.* My husband and I were both on board with healthier eating. Studies have shown that partner support in the ability to say no without wavering supports "healthy behavior."[158]
2. *Bribery.* Yes, I used healthier versions of their favorite foods (rice cereal and almond milk, for example) and rewarded their eating

a good meal with a treat afterward. This may or may not be the healthiest solution, but it helped our family.

3. *Better alternatives.* For school treats, birthday celebrations, or parties, I always had some allergen-free cookies, bars, or the like. I would also get gluten-free cupcakes from the local bakery for birthday parties. I always gave the teachers supplies to use during snack time or last minute birthdays so my children could have a special treat and not feel left out.

4. *Education.* Kids are extremely smart, and they do look up to you as parents for guidance. We talked a lot about the health reasons for why to choose an apple over a cookie. We also identified what their external response was to different food items. My middle child had had stomachaches and weird joint pains, and those went away when we ate well. We identified when high sugar was ingested that the kids "lost connection to their brain." We talked about it too. We talked about how they are smarter when they eat healthy and they can learn more. An added bonus was that my kids *love* learning, so it worked.

5. *Crowd-out principal.* Every meal we would offer plenty of healthy food so that they had options. If there were a few healthy items they actually liked, we had it readily available at every meal to a certain extent. If they fill up enough on the good stuff, then there won't be much room for the unhealthy stuff.

6. *Clean out the cupboards.* I have a real problem with self-control, so I can't expect my children to be better. I removed all packaged foods that had sugar, gluten, or trans-fatty acids. I donated them. It was hard-core, but the only way I knew our family wouldn't be tempted to eat it was to remove it. When I shop, I don't bring it home unless I plan on eating it.

7. *Make a plan.* Even today, when we go to a birthday party or BBQ, we talk about what is likely going to be available. They are allowed one juice box if available, not two, not three, and not four. We always bring something healthy to share. Funny how you rarely see vegetables or salads at parties anymore. We often eat before they go, so they don't find themselves starving when they arrive. It is easier to have self-control if your stomach is filled.

8. *Portion control.* I don't necessarily recommend this, but I did keep those special treats or things like maple syrup and ketchup in check. The kids do not have an endless supply of those, unlike fresh veggies and fruit.

9. *Surround yourself with likeminded people.* Fortunately for us, we have many friends who care about health and nutrition, so they welcome our kids into their homes. They love our kids eating salad, fruit, and vegetables and having a positive influence on their kids. I know this may be tricky for most, but sometimes taking a stand for your child allows others to take stands for their own children. The more you surround your kids with others who have similar eating habits, the more likely they will become like each other. [159] We all want to fit in.

10. *Don't be sneaky.* Trying to hide the healthy foods within an unhealthy item is not only deceptive, but also increases a parent's stress level and potentially produces a fussy eater.[158]

11. *Get the kids involved.* Letting kids take some ownership in the kitchen is possibly the most important step in getting children to eat healthy. We specifically have the kids make their own lunches, purely for sake of them owning their health. We are in control of what is available in the refrigerator, and they get to choose from there.

12. *Think outside the cracker box.* Avoiding gluten, for example, often leads to switching out wheat crackers for a "gluten-free" version. Although that is one way to avoid gluten, it certainly doesn't incorporate more nutrients. Thinking outside of the cracker/chip, replace with something whole that is also crunchy. For example, instead of crackers and cheese, try fresh cucumber, carrots, celery, or bell pepper slices and guacamole. For a twist with sweetness, try apple slices and nut butter with a sprinkle of cinnamon.

We never, *ever* made this about good or bad. Nor was it ever about weight control and appearance. It was *always* about health and feeding our body and brains what they needed most to be the healthiest as possible for school, for sports, for creativity, and for happiness. Like soar, there was a lot of variability and trial and error. Only you can know what best suits your child. I would say the first step is getting your partner on board, as that may be the most critical component. If you can't, then pick one component of nutrition and the KISS principles to work on. We ripped the Band-Aid off all at once, and certainly that will get you the most rapid results, but it isn't the only way. Any forward progress made is still progress, no matter how slow.

All parents feed their children food. No matter how you look at it, we are all spending time and money on the same activity. The different results lie solely on how we make our choices in what to eat.

Remove. Replace. Restore.

Remove passive parenting

Replace active involvement. Get the WHOLE family involved in the choices. Give healthy options and let individuals choose from there. Share information about why you make the choice, the children are listening.

Restore healthy growth.

Cost-Benefit Analysis

> Give a man a fish and you feed him for a day. Teach a man how to fish and you feed him for a lifetime.
>
> —Chinese proverb

I often get doubts about this lifestyle regarding the costs of organic meat and produce. Although I don't plan on sharing how much money we spend, I will say that I have found ways to make it more economical. These are the ways I see living this way saving us money:

1. We eat everything I buy and waste less food.
2. We eat out much less.
3. We buy bulk whenever possible to store or freeze.
4. We have less medical appointments, so fewer copays since we are sick less often.

The cheapest prices for nonperishable items are found online with shopping in bulk. Many stores have healthier food items available now, not just at the fancy markets, and sometimes for better prices too. Even bulk stores like Costco and Sam's Club have many great options for bulk organic produce and meats at good prices. Buying grass-fed meat is most available with the best prices from local farms. Here is a sample sign for standard eggs and organic eggs in a local bulk store. Notice that the cost is *only twenty* cents' different.

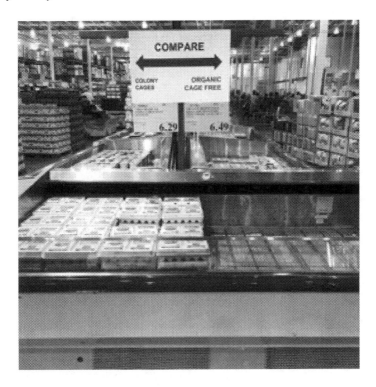

My job is to educate each patient so he or she can see how this lifestyle fits him or her. There are many means of saving money and planning meals whole foods–inspired, even on a budget. I believe it is not only possible but also necessary. Growing a backyard garden can also save you money. Where we spend our money as consumers is where the change is driven. All consumers need to be educated so they can be on alert for the booby traps too. KISS principles are for everyone to live by. Empowering every individual is the best way to achieving health. How we choose to spend our money is a personal decision, but as parents and health care providers, we must help others understand where they have control, regardless of financial and social status.

When someone tells me, "It is too expensive to eat whole foods" or "I can't afford to eat whole foods," I think one of three things: *can't, won't, or don't know how.* In the case of "can't," maybe they live in an area that doesn't provide any fresh-food items. I will admit that I can't help the problem directly if they don't have access to food or land to grow their own. I would argue that this is extremely rare, but it does exist. In the case of "won't," that person doesn't want to change, for they see no problem with their lives or health as it is. In this case, I can't change their minds, nor do I try. In order to make change, you have to first be open to it. In case of "don't know how," that becomes a window of opportunity, but it may require effort from the individual and an educator or health care provider. Sometimes people don't know how to improve their situations because they feel helpless.

I have come across many patients and even families who believe that they have no control over their situations. I include myself in this group until my journey started. This is called "learned helplessness," where an organism forced to endure aversive stimuli becomes unable or unwilling to avoid subsequent encounters, even if they are, in fact, escapable. The discovery of learned helplessness occurred accidentally in 1967 by Marin Seligman and Steven Maier in dogs. This helplessness can exacerbate several disorders, like depression, anxiety, phobias, shyness, and loneliness. Here is a schematic:

Undesirable event → Perceived lack of control → Generalized helplessness

In many cases, one can begin to expect a certain level of suffering. Just like a parent, a health care provider can educate and help lead someone to make a different choice to demonstrate he or she has control. It may not be that this lifestyle isn't affordable—because based on the eggs, I think it is—but rather someone doesn't know what the right choice is. Prior to my journey, I didn't *know* that what I was feeding children and myself was potentially making us sick. I had expected illness, as so many others around me went through similar things raising a family, dealing with depression, and gaining extra weight.

Exercise alone may have been my personal trigger to stimulate change in my lifestyle. As I exercised, it stimulated neuroplasticity that allowed me to feel a sense of well-being and happiness, and it even created new neural pathways that affected my behavior and thinking. [160] If you look at the details, eating *whole* foods is actually affordable; it just may not be what most know how to do. Rather than focusing on the monetary costs, maybe look at something that might help in learning new behaviors to escape learned helplessness, like exercise. Why don't we all take a walk in the sunshine to stimulate neuroplasticity so we can learn how to make better choices to support our health?

We may need to demonstrate positive change with not only exercise, but also time and education. It may not occur the first time, and it may take a few repetitions to actually change learned helplessness. Seligman demonstrated it took assisting the animals at least twice before they escaped the electrical shock and removed the learned helplessness behavior. [161] As parents and as health care providers, we owe it to our patients and to our children to keep trying. You never know which time will be the time that it actually effects the change. Keep trying until it does.

Remove. Replace. Restore.
Remove learned helplessness.
Replace education, exercise and repetition. It may take a few times, but as you move and try it will eventually drive the change.
Restore health.

Fad Turned Reality

If we could give every individual the right amount of nourishment and exercise, not too little and not too much, we would have found the safest way to healthy.

—Hippocrates

As my personal health journey progressed, I was extremely enthusiastic about the positive changes I was experiencing. I was so excited that I shared it too enthusiastically with anyone who was near me. I shared with other health care providers, nurses, and physicians. I shared it with family, including my parents, sister, brother, and cousins. I shared it with all my friends. It turns out that I made many people upset. I hurt their feelings. I am sorry for that. I wasn't trying to hurt anyone's feelings. I just wanted to share all this wonderful information with them so that they could have health too. I didn't realize how much emotion is tied in to food with guilt, shame, and connection.

Another pushback I got was related to the fad called the paleo diet. A fad, as defined by Merriam-Webster, is "something that many people are interested in for a short time; passing fashion; a craze." I would like to debunk this myth.

The word *paleo* may be a fad, but the information it represents is *not*. Whether or not you choose to believe in evolution or Paleolithic anthropology is your choice. The information regarding ideal human nutrition, movement, and sleep has been around for many years. In fact, Hippocrates, the father of Western medicine, had all these principles down way back in 460 BC. It is almost absurd how much scientific research there is in support of many of the principles and food recommendations that the paleo diet advocates. People like Loren Cordain, PhD, and Robb Wolf have brought the word *paleo* some publicity, but not because they discovered anything new. The information was there; they just put it in a format that made sense to us.

What makes the paleo "fad" different from most fitness and health-and-wellness fads, like P90X, Insanity, and the like, is that paleo's mission from the start has always been health, *not* a superficial goal of appearance of being a fitness or bikini model, not to mention that all their recommendations continue to be supported by the fundamentals of physiology, anatomy, and, yes, years and years of research. One goal is a moneymaking scheme, and one is a lifestyle change for health and disease prevention. Neither is all bad or all good; they are just different goals.

There have been times when I have had discussions with other PhD physical therapists, and I am surprised that they are so excited that I am thinking "outside the box." For me, I look at the KISS principles, and I see them all *inside* the box. We just forgot them because we were searching for proof or looking someplace else outside the box. What is outside of the box is medication, using viruses to cure brain cancer, diet soda, discovering something new about how our brain learns. How to eat, move, sleep and soar is not "outside the box." Think about it. What I write in this book is not really new at all. My message is simple. It is basic. It is fundamental. It is not a fad.

What we have on our hands as a community is not a fad but a movement of people who are looking for health. When I started this journey, I thought for sure more rapid change would happen. I felt I had just caught a wave of information just as it was peaking, and it would come crashing down into a revolution of change. That may or may not still happen. I am impatient. There are barriers. There is doubt, still.

I look forward to the day when we no longer fall prey to marketing schemes from the food industry, pharmaceutical industry, and fitness industry and simply learn how to care for ourselves within our communities. I look forward to when our children will thrive in all range of activities and learn without the bribery of sweets. I look forward to when the rates of autoimmune diseases like Parkinson's disease, multiple sclerosis, and the like plummet to nearly none. I look forward to watching my kids grow up healthy and have healthy children that I can enjoy when I am older. I look forward to when old means health and not disease. I look forward to the day when Western medicine is restored to health care and not sick care. I look forward to the day when the United States stands for health, that we don't bring sickness to other countries in the form of refined processed chemicals we call "food" in the name of goodwill.

When I look at those ideals, I need to pause. They are lofty ideals. I hope they aren't unrealistic perfection, but maybe they are. I am hopeful that improving your health is not only expected with following the KISS principles, but that it becomes a reality for you. I hope you continue to explore novel ways to attain health. Learn about the reasons why it works and share your story with me. Share your story with your loved ones. Share your story with your doctor or health care provider.

I have shared my story with you, and I look forward to hearing your story of health renewed. Soar into health with me.

Eat Well. Move Well. Sleep Well. Soar On.

Practicing Gratitude

There have been many people along the way who have supported me in this journey.

Thank you, dear Leah Williams. From afar, you supported, inspired, and kept me going. I wouldn't have continued this journey without your faith.

Thank you to the GiaQuinta family for making me feel like part of the family and inspiring me to continue writing.

Thank you to Grant Glass, PT, for starting this writing journey with me and supporting it with all your research and knowledge.

Thank you to fellow physical therapists Wendy Greene, Susan Pennington, and Danielle Litoff for starting this health journey with me. I am so glad to have other professionals and moms in my life to weed through the chaos.

Thank you to Kristine Richter for your help in starting my first business website. Your faith in me helped me make the first step.

Thank you to those who paved the way on the health movement. Your hard work and dedication continues to inspire and influence many. Robb Wolf, Loren Cordain, Sarah Ballantyne, Stacy and Matthew Toth, and Chris Kressor, by giving other clinicians something to share with patients and to continue to learn from, I am grateful.

Thank you to all those relentless scientists who need to continue to work to validate these principles in order to restore the order. Sorry we need you to work so hard, but thank you for your efforts.

Thank you to my gaggle of friends, family, and professionals who were willing to spare their precious time to give me input and edits on this book—Jamie Lindwall, Amy Conner, Leah Williams, Wendy Greene, Nancy Byl, Chris Dolan, Tara Finely, ND, Erich Krauss and Kristine Richter.

Thank you to all the staff at Author House publishing for keeping me on track and moving this project forward at a steady pace.

Thank you to my parents for showing me that there is more to life than just nutrition. Your love and support, although challenging at times, helped me in more ways than you will ever know.

Thank you to all my patients and clients for your trust, sharing your lives with me, and honoring me with the opportunity to help you recover so that you can soar.

Thank you to Chris, Ryan, Keenan, and Allison. You make my life a brighter place. I am blessed to have you in my life. I love you.

APPENDIX 1: SOAR KITCHEN STAPLES

Organic coconut flour
Organic almond flour
Tapioca or arrowroot flour
Coconut sugar
Coconut nectar (low-glycemic syrup alternative)
Coconut Aminos (soy sauce alternative, gluten-free)
Organic Cucina Antica ketchup (minimal sugar)
Organic maple sugar
Annie's Organic Yellow Mustard
Primal Kitchen Mayo with Avocado Oil (no trans-fatty acids—yahoo!)
Cold-pressed organic avocado oil (Chosen Foods)
Cold-pressed organic coconut oil (Spectrum)
Cold-pressed organic olive oil (Kirkland, Bragg)
Raw organic apple cider vinegar (Bragg's)
Organic balsamic vinegar (natural sulphites only!)
Kerrygold butter
Ghee (clarified butter)
Organic Cucina Antica spaghetti sauce (or others with no added sugars or preservatives)
Beef tallow (can be used for high heat cooking)
Great Lakes Gelatin

Full-fat coconut milk (Natural Value brand)
Almond/cashew milk (Pacifico brand organic)
Dark chocolate chips (Enjoy Life brand)
Organic vanilla (no additive or sugars)

APPENDIX 2: SOAR KITCHEN EQUIPMENT

High-speed blender (I use Vitamix)
Cast iron pan in two sizes
Nonstick pan
Firm BPA-free plastic spatula
Stainless steel spatula
Lemon squeezer
Spiralizer (for making zucchini noodles instead of pasta)
Waffle iron
Dehydrator
Mandolin (for evenly slicing root vegetables)
Crock-Pot Slow Cooker

APPENDIX 3: LATERAL SHIFT RECIPES

Better alternatives for when the "sweet tooth" strikes. These recipes are to be used occasionally and in addition to healthy whole foods nutrition.

Soar Jello

Serves 2-4

Ingredients:
16 ounces fresh-squeezed juice or *kombucha* (we love gingerade)
1/2 cup pure gelatin
1/2 cup boiling filtered water

Equipment:
High-speed blender
Glass Tupperware or Pyrex dish large enough to hold fluid (2-quart size total)
Measuring cup

Directions:
Prepare all ingredients and equipment prior to starting to mix ingredients. Once all equipment is ready, place the cold juice/kombucha in blender to

bring to room temperature. While waiting, mix the gelatin and hot water in large measuring cup until well combined. Then place in the blender and place top on the blender. Mix at high speed until well blended. This may take 60 seconds or more, depending on the temperature. Pour the mixture into the Pyrex or glass Tupperware. Cover and refrigerate for at least an hour or until thick. You can place in a mold to make it more interesting for children. Cut and enjoy as a treat, a snack, or a meal on the go.

(Inspired by Matthew and Stacy Toth from www.paleoparents.com)

Soar Movie Night Popcorn

Serves: 4-6

Ingredients:
1/4 cup organic coconut oil
2/3 cup organic, non-GMO corn kernels
2 tablespoons butter, melted
1 tablespoon raw honey or maple syrup
1 teaspoon sea salt

Equipment:
Large pot
Medium saucepan
Measuring cup
Measuring spoon
Rubber spatula

Directions:
Add the coconut oil and 3 kernels to the large pot. Cover and cook at medium heat until all kernels pop. Remove popped kernels and add the rest of the corn kernels. Cover and cook, shaking the pot intermittently until the popping slows. Remove from the heat and take the top off to keep crisp. While popping the corn, melt the butter in another pot and add the honey. Drizzle over the popcorn and mix. Sprinkle with salt. Serve and enjoy with a movie at home.

Soar "Ice Cream"

Serves:
2–4, depending

Ingredients:
2 frozen or room-temperature bananas
1 cup frozen organic berries of your choice
1/2 cup full-fat coconut milk/almond milk/cashew milk (preservative-free)
1–2 tablespoons of dark chocolate chips

Equipment:
High-speed blender
Measuring spoon
Measuring cup

Directions:
Place all ingredients into high-speed blender. Blend until smooth. If you have a masher tool with the blender, you will likely need it. Dish into small bowls and sprinkle with a few dark chocolate chips.

(Inspired by Michelle Tam and Henry Fong from *Nom Nom Paleo; Food for Humans*)

Soar "Pudding"

Serves:
2–4, depending

Ingredients:
2 frozen or room temperature bananas
1 ripe avocado
1/2 cup full fat coconut milk/almond milk/cashew milk (preservative-free)
1/4 cup organic powdered cocoa or cacao
1 tablespoon vanilla
1 teaspoon cinnamon

anti-inflammatory boost add 1 tablespoon turmeric

Equipment:
High-speed blender
Measuring spoon
Measuring cup

Directions:
Place all ingredients in the blender and puree until smooth. Return pudding into refrigerator until fully chilled. Top with fresh berries and enjoy.

(Inspired by Diane Sanfilippo in *Practical Paleo*)

Soar Frozen Banana Snacks

Serves:
4-6, depeding

Ingredients:
Whole bananas (how many you have determines how many you make)
1–2 tablespoons fresh almond butter (no additives or sugar, any nut or seed butter works)
1–2 tablespoons coconut chips
4–5 fresh berries, or as many as you have slices of bananas
1 teaspoon organic cinnamon

Equipment:
Small Pyrex dish with top (4x4) or small metal pan—anything that will fit into freezer
Wax paper

Directions:
Line your dish with wax paper. Cut the banana into 1/2-inch pieces that will lie flat in the dish. Top each banana slice with a bit of almond butter. Top with berry of your choice. Sprinkle the batch with coconut chips and sprinkle with cinnamon. Freeze until solid. Enjoy bite sized frozen banana bits. Skip freezing and enjoy as an afterschool snack.

Soar Spritzer

Serves: 1

Ingredients:
8 ounces carbonated water (I use a Sodastream to make carbonated filtered water at home.)
1 orange, lemon, or lime

Equipment:
Juicer (handheld)
Glass

Directions:
Add fresh-squeezed orange, lemon, or lime into carbonated water. Pour over ice and enjoy.

Soar Virgin Mimosa

Serves:
1-2

Ingredients:
8 ounces ginger kombucha
8 ounces fresh-squeezed organic orange juice

Directions:
Mix ingredients and serve. Enjoy.

Soar Spa Water

Serves:
1-2

Ingredients:
16 ounces fresh, filtered water
2–3 slices of organic cucumber, rinsed
1 sprig of organic mint, rinsed

Directions:
Place in the cucumber and mint with the water. Pour over ice and enjoy. You can switch out the cucumber and use any fruit you choose to make a more colorful drink.

Adult-Friendly Drink Alternative

"River Oaks"

Serves:
1-2

Ingredients:
8 ounces ginger kombucha (home brew or store-bought)
8 ounces fresh-squeezed organic orange juice
1 shot vodka (Tito's brand is gluten-free.)

Directions:
Mix ingredients and serve over ice. Enjoy on a sunny summer day with a good friend.

(In collaboration with Kristine Richter and Chris Dolan)

APPENDIX 4: SOAR FOUNDATIONAL RECIPES

Soar Salad Dressing

Ingredients:
1/2 cup olive oil/avocado oil or a mixture
1/2 cup vinegar (balsamic, apple cider, coconut, red wine—a mixture of whatever you have or are in the mood for)
Dash of organic yellow mustard
Dash of organic raw, local honey
Juice of 1 lemon

Directions:
Place all ingredients into a jar with a top. Shake vigorously and drizzle over your bed of greens. Mix equal parts of your oil of choice and vinegars of your choice. The only thing is to vary the ingredients regularly to find your favorite combination. If you want a creamier dressing, add an raw egg yolk if you have eggs from a trusted source.

(Inspired from my father, Fred Byl)

Soar Marinade

Ingredients:
1/2 yellow/white/red onion chopped
1/2 cup olive oil
1/2 cup balsamic vinegar
1/4 cup coconut aminos
2–3 chopped garlic cloves
1 tablespoon raw honey
1 teaspoon ground pepper
4 chicken breasts or equivalent protein

Directions:
Mix all ingredients and marinate your favorite protein for a few hours or overnight. It is good on pork, beef, or chicken.

(Inspired by making a paleo version of T-Linn special secret marinade)

APPENDIX 5: SOAR HEALING RECIPES

When healing, it is important to try to use organic ingredients to decrease the burden on the body, but these recipes are still extremely valuable even with standard ingredients. Be sure to carefully clean and peel all produce if using standard produce.

During healing it is important to continue with eating whole foods and to include more protein for the amino acids to help with repairing.

Soar Bone Broth

Ingredients:
1 whole, organic (free-range if possible) chicken carcass
Gizzards from one chicken (optional but increases nutrient richness)
1 beef long marrowbones if available from grass-fed and organic (optional but increases nutrient richness)
4 quarts filtered water, or enough to cover carcass in Crock-Pot
2 tablespoons vinegar
1 large organic onion, coarsely chopped
2–3 organic celery stalks, coarsely chopped
2 organic carrots, coarsely chopped
1 bunch organic parsley

Equipment:
Large 6-quart Crock-Pot with high and low settings
Knife
Cutting board
Large coarse strainer

Directions:
Place the chicken carcass, bones, and gizzards in Crock-Pot. Cover entirely with filtered water. You may need to add more water during the process. Add the vinegar and place Crock-Pot on low and relax. Simmer for up to 48 hours. For the last 4–6 hours, while bubbling, add the vegetables. Drain the contents through a strainer to catch the vegetables and carcass. Once the fluid cools, skim off the fat and reserve the stock in containers for use in soup and sauces or for drinking or traditional preparation of gluten-free grains. Can be stored in the freezer up to 6 moths. Can be stored in the refrigerator up to 5 days.

Soar Vegetable Broth

Ingredients:
2 organic, unpeeled whole carrots, roughly cut
2–3 organic garnet yam, red potato, or sweet potato, rinsed and roughly cut with skin on
1 medium organic yellow onion, roughly cut
1 bunch organic celery, roughly cut
1 bunch organic parsley
1 organic leek, roughly cut
2–4 cloves organic garlic, unpeeled and roughly cut in half
1 strip of kombu (sea vegetable)
1 teaspoon whole organic peppercorns
6–8 quarts filtered water
1/2 teaspoon sea salt or Herbamare (optional)

Equipment:
1 large stock pot (minimum 6-quart size, but bigger is better to fit all the vegetables)

Directions:
Rinse all vegetables and kombu. Roughly chop all vegetables. Place all ingredients except salt into the stockpot and cover with filtered water. Bring to a boil. Remove the lid and reduce to a simmer for 2–3 hours or until full flavor of the vegetables is smelled and tasted. Add the salt. Strain the stock through a large coarse strainer. Allow broth to come to room temperature before storing in the refrigerator or freezer. Can be stored in the freezer up to 6 months. Can be stored in the refrigerator up to 5 days. Use for soups, drinking, sauces, or traditional gluten-free grain preparations.

*Fiddle with the vegetable ingredients to your liking and preference and even seasonal availability.

APPENDIX 5: SOAR SNACK IDEAS

When there are birthdays, potlucks, games, and the like, these things keep our family going and are easy to bring and sometimes share.

Any whole fruit—tangerines, oranges, bananas, apples, pears
    Many stores offer precut fruits also for purchase.

Any whole vegetable—carrots, celery, snap peas
    Many stores offer precut veggies too, like jicama, celery, peppers, also for purchase.

Minimal ingredient bars—RxBar, Larabar, Rise Bar, Caveman, Cricket bar, Epic bar,
    That's It, Two-Moms
    These aren't perfect, but they do have options for either only natural sugar from fruit or close to five grams of added sugar. Look at the label.

APPENDIX 6: SOAR FOUNDATIONAL FLEXIBILITY

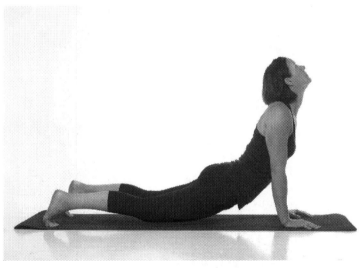

Extension in lying with neck extension

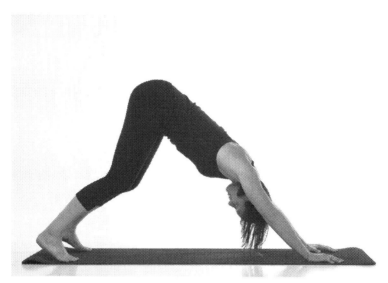

Downward dog pose modified for tight hamstrings. Can be done with full knee extension if have flexibility.

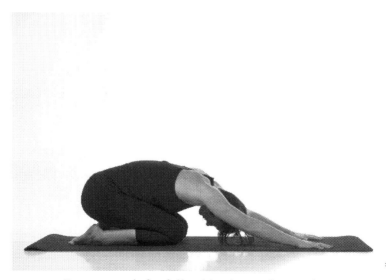

*

Prayer stretch for full ankle plantar flexion, knee flexion, shoulder flexion, and hip flexion.

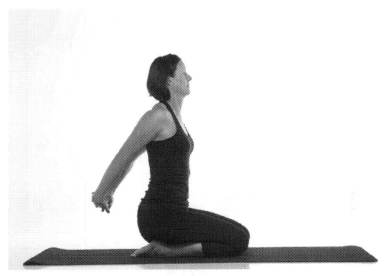

Kneeling shoulder extension. Can be done in standing or seated.

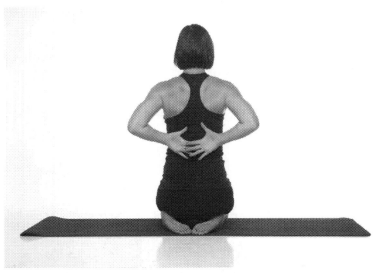

Kneeling shoulder internal rotation Can be done in standing or seated.

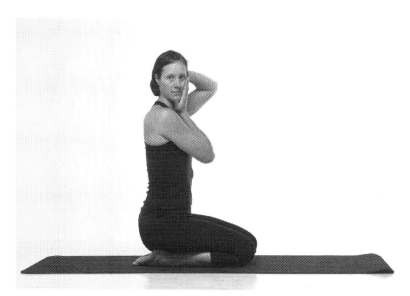

Cervical spine rotation with hand assist

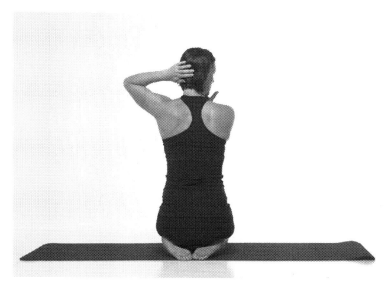

Cervical spine rotation with hand assist, posterior view

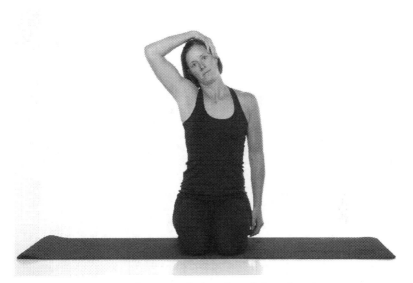

Cervical spine side bend with hand assist

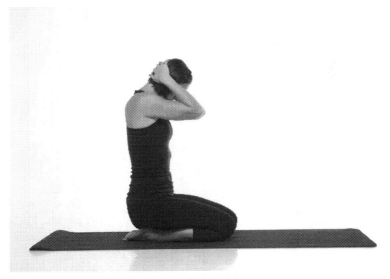

Cervical spine flexion with hands

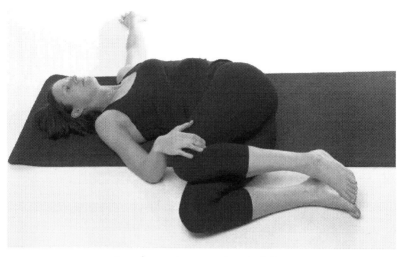

Lumbar spine rotation in lying

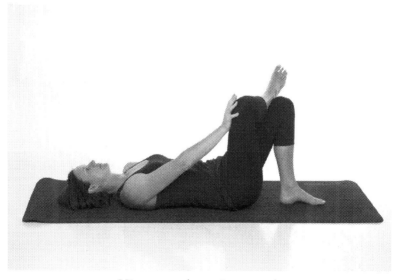

Hip external rotation stretch

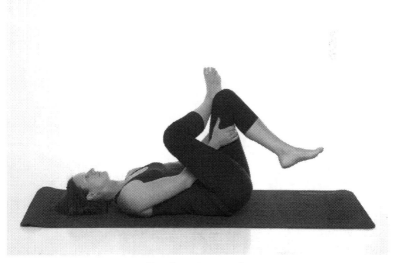

Piriformis stretch

APPENDIX 7: SOAR FOUNDATIONAL STRENGTHENING

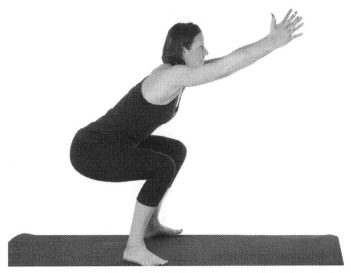

Squat with wide base of support, working hips below knees. Extend arms for balance and range of motion.

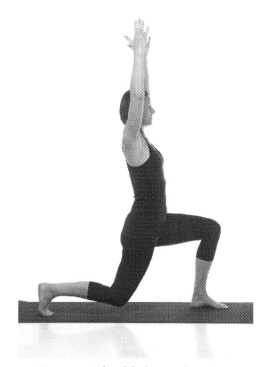

Lunges with added arm elevation.

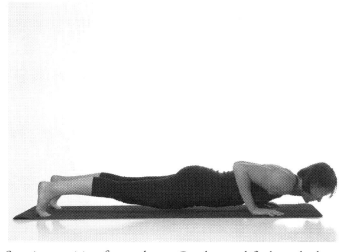

Starting position for push up. Can be modified on the knees.

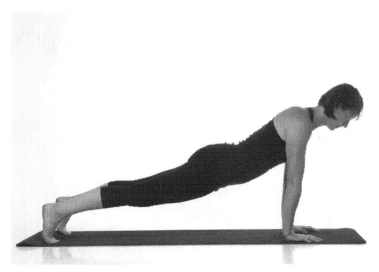

Ending position for push up.

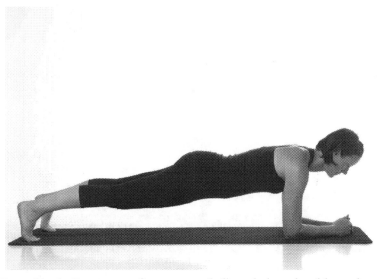

Front Plank: Resting on forearms and elbow below shoulders, elevate hips and hold as long as you can. Can be performed on knees.

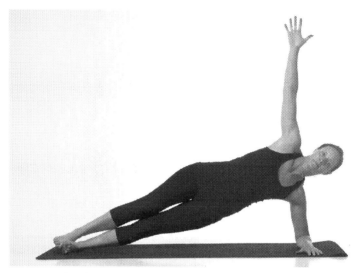

Side Plank: With elbow under shoulder, lift hips off
the floor and hold. Can be performed on knees.

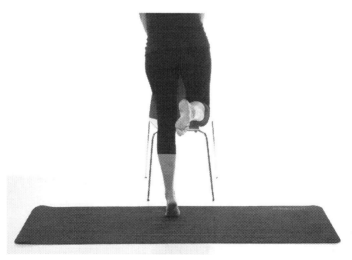

Single Heel Raise: Using a chair back or table to balance,
rise up onto toes, keeping forefoot on the ground.
Repeat as many as you can until fatigued.

NOTES

1. Neufeldt V, Guralnik D, eds. *Webster's new world dictionary of american english.* second ed. New York, New York: Webster's New World Dictionaries; 1988.

2. Mateljan G. *The world's healthiest foods.* First ed. Seattle, Washington: George Mateljan Foundation; 2007.

3. McGuire M, Beerman K, eds. *Nutritional sciences; from fundamentals to food.* Third Edition ed. Wadsworth; 2013.

4. Myers TM, Hoffman MD. Hiker fatality from severe hyponatremia in grand canyon national park. *Wilderness Environ Med.* 2015.

5. Hew-Butler T, Rosner MH, Fowkes-Godek S, et al. Statement of the third international exercise-associated hyponatremia consensus development conference, carlsbad, california, 2015. *Clin J Sport Med.* 2015;25(4):303-320.

6. Gandy J. Water intake: Validity of population assessment and recommendations. *Eur J Nutr.* 2015;54 Suppl 2:11-16.

7. Lipski, Elizabeth PhD CCn CHN. *Digestive wellness.* 4th Edition ed. United States of America: Mc GRaw Hill; 2012.

8. Branum AM, Lukacs SL. http://www.cdc.gov/nchs/data/databriefs/db10.htm#ref1.

9. Dickerson F, Stallings C, Origoni A, et al. Markers of gluten sensitivity and celiac disease in recent-onset psychosis and multi-episode schizophrenia. *Biol Psychiatry.* 2010;68(1):100-104.

10. Dickerson F, Stallings C, Origoni A, Vaughan C, Khushalani S, Yolken R. Markers of gluten sensitivity in acute mania: A longitudinal study. *Psychiatry Res.* 2012;196(1):68-71.

11. Dickerson F, Stallings C, Origoni A, et al. Markers of gluten sensitivity and celiac disease in bipolar disorder. *Bipolar Disord*. 2011;13(1):52-58.

12. Ben Abdelghani K, Mouelhi L, Hriz A, et al. Systemic lupus erythematosus and celiac disease. *Joint Bone Spine*. 2012;79(2):202-203.

13. Conti V, Leone MC, Casato M, Nicoli M, Granata G, Carlesimo M. High prevalence of gluten sensitivity in a cohort of patients with undifferentiated connective tissue disease. *Eur Ann Allergy Clin Immunol*. 2015;47(2):54-57.

14. Efe C, Purnak T, Ozaslan E, Ozbalkan Z. Back pain and sacroiliitis in long-standing adult celiac disease: A cross-sectional and follow-up study. *Rheumatol Int*. 2011;31(2):279-010-1375-8. Epub 2010 Feb 20.

15. Lerner A, Matthias T. Rheumatoid arthritis-celiac disease relationship: Joints get that gut feeling. *Autoimmun Rev*. 2015.

16. Togrol RE, Nalbant S, Solmazgul E, et al. The significance of coeliac disease antibodies in patients with ankylosing spondylitis: A case-controlled study. *J Int Med Res*. 2009;37(1):220-226.

17. Ozyemisci-Taskiran O, Cengiz M, Atalay F. Celiac disease of the joint. *Rheumatol Int*. 2011;31(5):573-576.

18. Hu Y, Costenbader KH, Gao X, et al. Sugar-sweetened soda consumption and risk of developing rheumatoid arthritis in women. *Am J Clin Nutr*. 2014;100(3):959-967.

19. Guo X, Park Y, Freedman ND, et al. Sweetened beverages, coffee, and tea and depression risk among older US adults. *PLoS One*. 2014;9(4):e94715.

20. Sellam J, Berenbaum F. Is osteoarthritis a metabolic disease? *Joint Bone Spine*. 2013;80(6):568-573.

21. Sanchez A, Reeser JL, Lau HS, et al. Role of sugars in human neutrophilic phagocytosis. *Am J Clin Nutr*. 1973;26(11):1180-1184.

22. Jungmann PM, Kraus MS, Alizai H, et al. Association of metabolic risk factors with cartilage degradation assessed by T2 relaxation time at the knee: Data from the osteoarthritis initiative. *Arthritis Care Res (Hoboken)*. 2013;65(12):1942-1950.

23. Aquilani R, Boselli M, Paola B, et al. Is stroke rehabilitation a metabolic problem? *Brain Inj*. 2014;28(2):161-173.

24. Lindmeier C. http://www.who.int/mediacentre/news/releases/2015/sugar-guideline/en/.

25. Suez J, Korem T, Zeevi D, et al. Artificial sweeteners induce glucose intolerance by altering the gut microbiota. *Nature*. 2014;514(7521):181-186.

26. Bendsen NT, Christensen R, Bartels EM, Astrup A. Consumption of industrial and ruminant trans fatty acids and risk of coronary heart disease: A systematic review and meta-analysis of cohort studies. *Eur J Clin Nutr*. 2011;65(7):773-783.

27. Trevizol F, Roversi K, Dias VT, et al. Cross-generational trans fat intake facilitates mania-like behavior: Oxidative and molecular markers in brain cortex. *Neuroscience*. 2015;286:353-363.

28. Barcelos RC, Vey LT, Segat HJ, et al. Cross-generational trans fat intake exacerbates UV radiation-induced damage in rat skin. *Food Chem Toxicol.* 2014;69:38-45.

29. Nestel P. Trans fatty acids: Are its cardiovascular risks fully appreciated? *Clin Ther.* 2014;36(3):315-321.

30. Lingelbach LB, Mitchell AE, Rucker RB, McDonald RB. Accumulation of advanced glycation endproducts in aging male fischer 344 rats during long-term feeding of various dietary carbohydrates. *J Nutr.* 2000;130(5):1247-1255.

31. Li Y, Fessel G, Georgiadis M, Snedeker JG. Advanced glycation end-products diminish tendon collagen fiber sliding. *Matrix Biol.* 2013;32(3-4):169-177.

32. Spreadbury I. Comparison with ancestral diets suggests dense acellular carbohydrates promote an inflammatory microbiota, and may be the primary dietary cause of leptin resistance and obesity. *Diabetes Metab Syndr Obes.* 2012;5:175-189.

33. Ruskin DN, Kawamura M, Masino SA. Reduced pain and inflammation in juvenile and adult rats fed a ketogenic diet. *PLoS One.* 2009;4(12):e8349.

34. Chen Y, Fan JX, Zhang ZL, et al. The negative influence of high-glucose ambience on neurogenesis in developing quail embryos. *PLoS One.* 2013;8(6):e66646.

35. Rodrigues DF, Henriques MC, Oliveira MC, et al. Acute intake of a high-fructose diet alters the balance of adipokine concentrations and induces neutrophil influx in the liver. *J Nutr Biochem.* 2014;25(4):388-394.

36. Mikulikova K, Eckhardt A, Kunes J, Zicha J, Miksik I. Advanced glycation end-product pentosidine accumulates in various tissues of rats with high fructose intake. *Physiol Res.* 2008;57(1):89-94.

37. Felice JI, Gangoiti MV, Molinuevo MS, McCarthy AD, Cortizo AM. Effects of a metabolic syndrome induced by a fructose-rich diet on bone metabolism in rats. *Metabolism.* 2014;63(2):296-305.

38. Robbins PI, Raymond L. Aspartame and symptoms of carpal tunnel syndrome. *J Occup Environ Med.* 1999;41(6):418.

39. Horio Y, Sun Y, Liu C, Saito T, Kurasaki M. Aspartame-induced apoptosis in PC12 cells. *Environ Toxicol Pharmacol.* 2014;37(1):158-165.

40. Ashok I, Sheeladevi R. Biochemical responses and mitochondrial mediated activation of apoptosis on long-term effect of aspartame in rat brain. *Redox Biol.* 2014;2:820-831.

41. Abdel-Salam OM, Salem NA, El-Shamarka ME, Hussein JS, Ahmed NA, El-Nagar ME. Studies on the effects of aspartame on memory and oxidative stress in brain of mice. *Eur Rev Med Pharmacol Sci.* 2012;16(15):2092-2101.

42. Suez J, Korem T, Zeevi D, et al. Artificial sweeteners induce glucose intolerance by altering the gut microbiota. *Nature.* 2014;514(7521):181-186.

43. Lindseth GN, Coolahan SE, Petros TV, Lindseth PD. Neurobehavioral effects of aspartame consumption. *Res Nurs Health.* 2014;37(3):185-193.

44. Rycerz K, Jaworska-Adamu JE. Effects of aspartame metabolites on astrocytes and neurons. *Folia Neuropathol.* 2013;51(1):10-17.

45. Alkafafy ME, Ibrahim ZS, Ahmed MM, El-Shazly SA. Impact of aspartame and saccharin on the rat liver: Biochemical, molecular, and histological approach. *Int J Immunopathol Pharmacol.* 2015.

46. Karl JP, Alemany JA, Koenig C, et al. Diet, body composition, and physical fitness influences on IGF-I bioactivity in women. *Growth Horm IGF Res.* 2009;19(6):491-496.

47. Baad-Hansen L, Cairns B, Ernberg M, Svensson P. Effect of systemic monosodium glutamate (MSG) on headache and pericranial muscle sensitivity. *Cephalalgia.* 2010;30(1):68-76.

48. Shimada A, Cairns BE, Vad N, et al. Headache and mechanical sensitization of human pericranial muscles after repeated intake of monosodium glutamate (MSG). *J Headache Pain.* 2013;14(1):2-2377-14-2.

49. Bernardo D, Garrote JA, Fernandez-Salazar L, Riestra S, Arranz E. Is gliadin really safe for non-coeliac individuals? production of interleukin 15 in biopsy culture from non-coeliac individuals challenged with gliadin peptides. *Gut.* 2007;56(6):889-890.

50. de Oliveira LP, Vieira CP, Da Re Guerra F, de Almeida Mdos S, Pimentel ER. Statins induce biochemical changes in the achilles tendon after chronic treatment. *Toxicology.* 2013;311(3):162-168.

51. Chechik O, Dolkart O, Mozes G, Rak O, Alhajajra F, Maman E. Timing matters: NSAIDs interfere with the late proliferation stage of a repaired rotator cuff tendon healing in rats. *Arch Orthop Trauma Surg.* 2014;134(4):515-520.

52. Berg AM, Dam AN, Farraye FA. Environmental influences on the onset and clinical course of crohn's disease-part 2: Infections and medication use. *Gastroenterol Hepatol (N Y).* 2013;9(12):803-810.

53. Dam AN, Berg AM, Farraye FA. Environmental influences on the onset and clinical course of crohn's disease-part 1: An overview of external risk factors. *Gastroenterol Hepatol (N Y).* 2013;9(11):711-717.

54. Blackmore KM, Wong J, Knight JA. A cross-sectional study of different patterns of oral contraceptive use among premenopausal women and circulating IGF-1: Implications for disease risk. *BMC Womens Health.* 2011;11:15-6874-11-15.

55. Okada Y, Tsuzuki Y, Ueda T, et al. Trans fatty acids in diets act as a precipitating factor for gut inflammation? *J Gastroenterol Hepatol.* 2013;28 Suppl 4:29-32.

56. Ahmad SO, Park JH, Radel JD, Levant B. Reduced numbers of dopamine neurons in the substantia nigra pars compacta and ventral tegmental area of rats fed an n-3 polyunsaturated fatty acid-deficient diet: A stereological study. *Neurosci Lett.* 2008;438(3):303-307.

57. Grasa J, Calvo B, Delgado-Andrade C, Navarro MP. Variations in tendon stiffness due to diets with different glycotoxins affect mechanical properties in the muscle-tendon unit. *Ann Biomed Eng.* 2013;41(3):488-496.

58. Bisht B, Darling WG, Grossmann RE, et al. A multimodal intervention for patients with secondary progressive multiple sclerosis: Feasibility and effect on fatigue. *J Altern Complement Med.* 2014;20(5):347-355.

59. Pottenger FM. *Pottenger's cats: A study in nutrition.* Second Edition ed. Lemon Grove, CA: Price-Pottenger Nutrition Foundation, Inc; 2012.

60. Shulman RJ, Jarrett ME, Cain KC, Broussard EK, Heitkemper MM. Associations among gut permeability, inflammatory markers, and symptoms in patients with irritable bowel syndrome. *J Gastroenterol.* 2014;49(11):1467-1476.

61. Samaroo D, Dickerson F, Kasarda DD, et al. Novel immune response to gluten in individuals with schizophrenia. *Schizophr Res.* 2010;118(1-3):248-255.

62. Dickerson FB, Stallings C, Origoni A, et al. Effect of probiotic supplementation on schizophrenia symptoms and association with gastrointestinal functioning: A randomized, placebo-controlled trial. *Prim Care Companion CNS Disord.* 2014;16(1):10.4088/PCC.13m01579. Epub 2014 Feb 13.

63. Giardina S, Scilironi C, Michelotti A, et al. In vitro anti-inflammatory activity of selected oxalate-degrading probiotic bacteria: Potential applications in the prevention and treatment of hyperoxaluria. *J Food Sci.* 2014;79(3):M384-90.

64. Berg AM, Dam AN, Farraye FA. Environmental influences on the onset and clinical course of crohn's disease-part 2: Infections and medication use. *Gastroenterol Hepatol (N Y).* 2013;9(12):803-810.

65. Rheaume-Bleue KN. *Vitamin K2 and the calcium paradox; how A little-known vitamin could save your life.* Toronto, Ontario, Canada: Harper Collins Publisher; 2012.

66. Poloni A, Maurizi G, Anastasi S, et al. Plasticity of human dedifferentiated adipocytes toward endothelial cells. *Exp Hematol.* 2015;43(2):137-146.

67. Giordano A, Smorlesi A, Frontini A, Barbatelli G, Cinti S. White, brown and pink adipocytes: The extraordinary plasticity of the adipose organ. *Eur J Endocrinol.* 2014;170(5):R159-71.

68. Tholpady SS, Aojanepong C, Llull R, et al. The cellular plasticity of human adipocytes. *Ann Plast Surg.* 2005;54(6):651-656.

69. Marques CG, Santos VC, Levada-Pires AC, et al. Effects of DHA-rich fish oil supplementation on the lipid profile, markers of muscle damage, and neutrophil function in wheelchair basketball athletes before and after acute exercise. *Appl Physiol Nutr Metab.* 2015:1-9.

70. Venturini D, Simao AN, Urbano MR, Dichi I. Effects of extra virgin olive oil and fish oil on lipid profile and oxidative stress in patients with metabolic syndrome. *Nutrition.* 2015;31(6):834-840.

71. Badr G, Badr BM, Mahmoud MH, Mohany M, Rabah DM, Garraud O. Treatment of diabetic mice with undenatured whey protein accelerates the wound healing process by enhancing the expression of MIP-1alpha, MIP-2, KC, CX3CL1 and TGF-beta in wounded tissue. *BMC Immunol.* 2012;13:32-2172-13-32.

72. Badr G. Camel whey protein enhances diabetic wound healing in a streptozotocin-induced diabetic mouse model: The critical role of beta-defensin-1, -2 and -3. *Lipids Health Dis.* 2013;12:46-511X-12-46.

73. Badr G, Badr BM, Mahmoud MH, Mohany M, Rabah DM, Garraud O. Treatment of diabetic mice with undenatured whey protein accelerates the wound healing process by enhancing the expression of MIP-1alpha, MIP-2, KC, CX3CL1 and TGF-beta in wounded tissue. *BMC Immunol.* 2012;13:32-2172-13-32.

74. Badr G. Supplementation with undenatured whey protein during diabetes mellitus improves the healing and closure of diabetic wounds through the rescue of functional long-lived wound macrophages. *Cell Physiol Biochem.* 2012;29(3-4):571-582.

75. Ebaid H, Ahmed OM, Mahmoud AM, Ahmed RR. Limiting prolonged inflammation during proliferation and remodeling phases of wound healing in streptozotocin-induced diabetic rats supplemented with camel undenatured whey protein. *BMC Immunol.* 2013;14:31-2172-14-31.

76. Ebaid H, Salem A, Sayed A, Metwalli A. Whey protein enhances normal inflammatory responses during cutaneous wound healing in diabetic rats. *Lipids Health Dis.* 2011;10:235-511X-10-235.

77. Oner OZ, Ogunc AV, Cingi A, Uyar SB, Yalcin AS, Aktan AO. Whey feeding suppresses the measurement of oxidative stress in experimental burn injury. *Surg Today.* 2006;36(4):376-381.

78. Daly RM, O'Connell SL, Mundell NL, Grimes CA, Dunstan DW, Nowson CA. Protein-enriched diet, with the use of lean red meat, combined with progressive resistance training enhances lean tissue mass and muscle strength and reduces circulating IL-6 concentrations in elderly women: A cluster randomized controlled trial. *Am J Clin Nutr.* 2014;99(4):899-910.

79. Han Q, Yang P, Wu Y, et al. Epigenetically modified bone marrow stromal cells (BMSCs) in silk scaffolds promote craniofacial bone repair and wound healing. *Tissue Eng Part A.* 2015.

80. Hu Y, Costenbader KH, Gao X, et al. Sugar-sweetened soda consumption and risk of developing rheumatoid arthritis in women. *Am J Clin Nutr.* 2014;100(3):959-967.

81. Xiao S, Fei N, Pang X, et al. A gut microbiota-targeted dietary intervention for amelioration of chronic inflammation underlying metabolic syndrome. *FEMS Microbiol Ecol.* 2014;87(2):357-367.

82. Vaghef-Mehrabany E, Alipour B, Homayouni-Rad A, Sharif SK, Asghari-Jafarabadi M, Zavvari S. Probiotic supplementation improves inflammatory status in patients with rheumatoid arthritis. *Nutrition*. 2014;30(4):430-435.

83. Barbosa AW, Benevides GP, Alferes LM, Salomao EM, Gomes-Marcondes MC, Gomes L. A leucine-rich diet and exercise affect the biomechanical characteristics of the digital flexor tendon in rats after nutritional recovery. *Amino Acids*. 2012;42(1):329-336.

84. Takeuchi H, Kondo Y, Yanagi M, Yoshikawa M. Accelerative effect of olive oil on adrenal corticosterone secretion in rats loaded with single or repetitive immersion-restraint stress. *J Nutr Sci Vitaminol (Tokyo)*. 2000;46(4):158-164.

85. Takeuchi H, Suzuki N, Tada M, He P. Accelerative effect of olive oil on liver glycogen synthesis in rats subjected to water-immersion restraint stress. *Biosci Biotechnol Biochem*. 2001;65(7):1489-1494.

86. Atiba A, Nishimura M, Kakinuma S, et al. Aloe vera oral administration accelerates acute radiation-delayed wound healing by stimulating transforming growth factor-beta and fibroblast growth factor production. *Am J Surg*. 2011;201(6):809-818.

87. Ao J, Li B. Amino acid composition and antioxidant activities of hydrolysates and peptide fractions from porcine collagen. *Food Sci Technol Int*. 2012;18(5):425-434.

88. Liu J, Peter K, Shi D, et al. Anti-inflammatory effects of the chinese herbal formula sini tang in myocardial infarction rats. *Evid Based Complement Alternat Med*. 2014;2014:309378.

89. San Miguel SM, Opperman LA, Allen EP, Zielinski JE, Svoboda KK. Antioxidant combinations protect oral fibroblasts against metal-induced toxicity. *Arch Oral Biol*. 2013;58(3):299-310.

90. Urios P, Grigorova-Borsos AM, Sternberg M. Flavonoids inhibit the formation of the cross-linking AGE pentosidine in collagen incubated with glucose, according to their structure. *Eur J Nutr*. 2007;46(3):139-146.

91. Kim RJ, Hah YS, Sung CM, Kang JR, Park HB. Do antioxidants inhibit oxidative-stress-induced autophagy of tenofibroblasts? *J Orthop Res*. 2014.

92. Demirkol A, Uludag M, Soran N, et al. Total oxidative stress and antioxidant status in patients with carpal tunnel syndrome. *Redox Rep*. 2012;17(6):234-238.

93. Park HB, Hah YS, Yang JW, Nam JB, Cho SH, Jeong ST. Antiapoptotic effects of anthocyanins on rotator cuff tenofibroblasts. *J Orthop Res*. 2010;28(9):1162-1169.

94. Grieger JA, Wood LG, Clifton VL. Antioxidant-rich dietary intervention for improving asthma control in pregnancies complicated by asthma: Study protocol for a randomized controlled trial. *Trials*. 2014;15:108-6215-15-108.

95. Baez-Saldana A, Gutierrez-Ospina G, Chimal-Monroy J, Fernandez-Mejia C, Saavedra R. Biotin deficiency in mice is associated with decreased serum availability of insulin-like growth factor-I. *Eur J Nutr*. 2009;48(3):137-144.

96. Playford RJ, Floyd DN, Macdonald CE, et al. Bovine colostrum is a health food supplement which prevents NSAID induced gut damage. *Gut.* 1999;44(5):653-658.

97. Colpo E, Dalton D A Vilanova C, Reetz LG, et al. Brazilian nut consumption by healthy volunteers improves inflammatory parameters. *Nutrition.* 2014;30(4):459-465.

98. Kim J, Jeong IH, Kim CS, Lee YM, Kim JM, Kim JS. Chlorogenic acid inhibits the formation of advanced glycation end products and associated protein cross-linking. *Arch Pharm Res.* 2011;34(3):495-500.

99. Busch F, Mobasheri A, Shayan P, Lueders C, Stahlmann R, Shakibaei M. Resveratrol modulates interleukin-1beta-induced phosphatidylinositol 3-kinase and nuclear factor kappaB signaling pathways in human tenocytes. *J Biol Chem.* 2012;287(45):38050-38063.

100. Cho KS, Lee EJ, Kwon KJ, et al. Resveratrol down-regulates a glutamate-induced tissue plasminogen activator via erk and AMPK/mTOR pathways in rat primary cortical neurons. *Food Funct.* 2014;5(5):951-960.

101. Gordon BS, Delgado-Diaz DC, Carson J, Fayad R, Wilson LB, Kostek MC. Resveratrol improves muscle function but not oxidative capacity in young mdx mice. *Can J Physiol Pharmacol.* 2014;92(3):243-251.

102. Lei M, Wang JG, Xiao DM, et al. Resveratrol inhibits interleukin 1beta-mediated inducible nitric oxide synthase expression in articular chondrocytes by activating SIRT1 and thereby suppressing nuclear factor-kappaB activity. *Eur J Pharmacol.* 2012;674(2-3):73-79.

103. Yang SJ, Lim Y. Resveratrol ameliorates hepatic metaflammation and inhibits NLRP3 inflammasome activation. *Metabolism.* 2014;63(5):693-701.

104. Liu FC, Hung LF, Wu WL, et al. Chondroprotective effects and mechanisms of resveratrol in advanced glycation end products-stimulated chondrocytes. *Arthritis Res Ther.* 2010;12(5):R167.

105. Shakibaei M, Mobasheri A, Buhrmann C. Curcumin synergizes with resveratrol to stimulate the MAPK signaling pathway in human articular chondrocytes in vitro. *Genes Nutr.* 2011;6(2):171-179.

106. Somchit M, Changtam C, Kimseng R, et al. Demethoxycurcumin from curcuma longa rhizome suppresses iNOS induction in an in vitro inflamed human intestinal mucosa model. *Asian Pac J Cancer Prev.* 2014;15(4):1807-1810.

107. Ganjali S, Sahebkar A, Mahdipour E, et al. Investigation of the effects of curcumin on serum cytokines in obese individuals: A randomized controlled trial. *ScientificWorldJournal.* 2014;2014:898361.

108. Gomez-Pinilla F, Tyagi E. Diet and cognition: Interplay between cell metabolism and neuronal plasticity. *Curr Opin Clin Nutr Metab Care.* 2013;16(6):726-733.

109. Dawson DR,3rd, Branch-Mays G, Gonzalez OA, Ebersole JL. Dietary modulation of the inflammatory cascade. *Periodontol 2000.* 2014;64(1):161-197.

110. Kaminski WE, Jendraschak E, Kiefl R, von Schacky C. Dietary omega-3 fatty acids lower levels of platelet-derived growth factor mRNA in human mononuclear cells. *Blood.* 1993;81(7):1871-1879.

111. Silva PS, Sperandio da Silva GM, de Souza AP, et al. Effects of omega-3 polyunsaturated fatty acid supplementation in patients with chronic chagasic cardiomyopathy: Study protocol for a randomized controlled trial. *Trials.* 2013;14:379-6215-14-379.

112. Passos PP, Borba JM, Rocha-de-Melo AP, et al. Dopaminergic cell populations of the rat substantia nigra are differentially affected by essential fatty acid dietary restriction over two generations. *J Chem Neuroanat.* 2012;44(2):66-75.

113. Hansen RA, Harris MA, Pluhar GE, et al. Fish oil decreases matrix metalloproteinases in knee synovia of dogs with inflammatory joint disease. *J Nutr Biochem.* 2008;19(2):101-108.

114. Lionetti L, Mollica MP, Sica R, et al. Differential effects of high-fish oil and high-lard diets on cells and cytokines involved in the inflammatory process in rat insulin-sensitive tissues. *Int J Mol Sci.* 2014;15(2):3040-3063.

115. Wei HK, Zhou Y, Jiang S, et al. Feeding a DHA-enriched diet increases skeletal muscle protein synthesis in growing pigs: Association with increased skeletal muscle insulin action and local mRNA expression of insulin-like growth factor 1. *Br J Nutr.* 2013;110(4):671-680.

116. Luo C, Ren H, Wan JB, et al. Enriched endogenous omega-3 fatty acids in mice protect against global ischemia injury. *J Lipid Res.* 2014;55(7):1288-1297.

117. Cardoso HD, Passos PP, Lagranha CJ, et al. Differential vulnerability of substantia nigra and corpus striatum to oxidative insult induced by reduced dietary levels of essential fatty acids. *Front Hum Neurosci.* 2012;6:249.

118. Cardoso HD, dos Santos Junior EF, de Santana DF, et al. Omega-3 deficiency and neurodegeneration in the substantia nigra: Involvement of increased nitric oxide production and reduced BDNF expression. *Biochim Biophys Acta.* 2014;1840(6):1902-1912.

119. McCarty MF, Barroso-Aranda J, Contreras F. Potential complementarity of high-flavanol cocoa powder and spirulina for health protection. *Med Hypotheses.* 2010;74(2):370-373.

120. Gu Y, Yu S, Park JY, Harvatine K, Lambert JD. Dietary cocoa reduces metabolic endotoxemia and adipose tissue inflammation in high-fat fed mice. *J Nutr Biochem.* 2014;25(4):439-445.

121. Laparra JM, Lopez-Rubio A, Lagaron JM, Sanz Y. Dietary glycosaminoglycans interfere in bacterial adhesion and gliadin-induced pro-inflammatory response in intestinal epithelial (caco-2) cells. *Int J Biol Macromol.* 2010;47(4):458-464.

122. Carames B, Kiosses WB, Akasaki Y, et al. Glucosamine activates autophagy in vitro and in vivo. *Arthritis Rheum.* 2013;65(7):1843-1852.

123. Angeline ME, Ma R, Pascual-Garrido C, et al. Effect of diet-induced vitamin D deficiency on rotator cuff healing in a rat model. *Am J Sports Med.* 2014;42(1):27-34.

124. Park YE, Kim BH, Lee SG, et al. Vitamin D status of patients with early inflammatory arthritis. *Clin Rheumatol.* 2014.

125. Sanghi D, Mishra A, Sharma AC, et al. Does vitamin D improve osteoarthritis of the knee: A randomized controlled pilot trial. *Clin Orthop Relat Res.* 2013;471(11):3556-3562.

126. Baggerly CA, Cuomo RE, French CB, et al. Sunlight and vitamin D: Necessary for public health. *J Am Coll Nutr.* 2015;34(4):359-365.

127. Park KY, Chung PW, Kim YB, et al. Serum vitamin D status as a predictor of prognosis in patients with acute ischemic stroke. *Cerebrovasc Dis.* 2015;40(1-2):73-80.

128. Bachstetter AD, Jernberg J, Schlunk A, et al. Spirulina promotes stem cell genesis and protects against LPS induced declines in neural stem cell proliferation. *PLoS One.* 2010;5(5):e10496.

129. Ryan MJ, Dudash HJ, Docherty M, et al. Vitamin E and C supplementation reduces oxidative stress, improves antioxidant enzymes and positive muscle work in chronically loaded muscles of aged rats. *Exp Gerontol.* 2010;45(11):882-895.

130. Hung LK, Fu SC, Lee YW, Mok TY, Chan KM. Local vitamin-C injection reduced tendon adhesion in a chicken model of flexor digitorum profundus tendon injury. *J Bone Joint Surg Am.* 2013;95(7):e41.

131. Benoit B, Plaisancie P, Geloen A, et al. Pasture v. standard dairy cream in high-fat diet-fed mice: Improved metabolic outcomes and stronger intestinal barrier. *Br J Nutr.* 2014;112(4):520-535.

132. Bordoni A, Danesi F, Dardevet D, et al. Dairy products and inflammation: A review of the clinical evidence. *Crit Rev Food Sci Nutr.* 2015:0.

133. Lee HS, Park SY, Park Y, Bae SH, Suh HJ. Yeast hydrolysate protects cartilage via stimulation of type II collagen synthesis and suppression of MMP-13 production. *Phytother Res.* 2013;27(9):1414-1418.

134. Liu S, Willett WC, Stampfer MJ, et al. A prospective study of dietary glycemic load, carbohydrate intake, and risk of coronary heart disease in US women. *Am J Clin Nutr.* 2000;71(6):1455-1461.

135. Campbell B, Wilborn C, La Bounty P, et al. International society of sports nutrition position stand: Energy drinks. *J Int Soc Sports Nutr.* 2013;10(1):1-2783-10-1.

136. Lawford BJ, Walters J, Ferrar K. Does walking improve disability status, function, or quality of life in adults with chronic low back pain? A systematic review. *Clin Rehabil.* 2015.

137. Monteiro-Junior RS, Cevada T, Oliveira BR, et al. We need to move more: Neurobiological hypotheses of physical exercise as a treatment for parkinson's disease. *Med Hypotheses.* 2015.

138. Greenwood BN, Fleshner M. Exercise, stress resistance, and central serotonergic systems. *Exerc Sport Sci Rev.* 2011;39(3):140-149.

139. Wicker P, Frick B. The relationship between intensity and duration of physical activity and subjective well-being. *Eur J Public Health.* 2015.

140. Arnardottir NY, Koster A, Domelen DR, et al. Association of change in brain structure to objectively measured physical activity and sedentary behavior in older adults: Age, gene/environment susceptibility-reykjavik study. *Behav Brain Res.* 2015;296:118-124.

141. Stewart RA, Benatar J, Maddison R. Living longer by sitting less and moving more. *Curr Opin Cardiol.* 2015;30(5):551-557.

142. Bergland A, Laake K. Concurrent and predictive validity of "getting up from lying on the floor". *Aging Clin Exp Res.* 2005;17(3):181-185.

143. Healy GN, Winkler EA, Owen N, Anuradha S, Dunstan DW. Replacing sitting time with standing or stepping: Associations with cardio-metabolic risk biomarkers. *Eur Heart J.* 2015.

144. Prior J, Bauman A, Ding M, et al. Sedentary behaviour, sitting and mortality-cross-sectional and 10 y prospective data. 2015.

145. Fallon S, Enig M. *Nourishing traditions; the cookbook that challenges politically correct nutrition and the diet dictocrats.* Brandywine, MD: NewTrends Publishing, Inc; 2001.

146. Lieberman S, Bruning N. *The real vitamin and mineral book.* New York, New York: The Penguin Group; 2007.

147. Park YE, Kim BH, Lee SG, et al. Vitamin D status of patients with early inflammatory arthritis. *Clin Rheumatol.* 2015;34(2):239-246.

148. Broder AR, Tobin JN, Putterman C. Disease-specific definitions of vitamin D deficiency need to be established in autoimmune and non-autoimmune chronic diseases: A retrospective comparison of three chronic diseases. *Arthritis Res Ther.* 2010;12(5):R191.

149. Terushkin V, Bender A, Psaty EL, Engelsen O, Wang SQ, Halpern AC. Estimated equivalency of vitamin D production from natural sun exposure versus oral vitamin D supplementation across seasons at two US latitudes. *J Am Acad Dermatol.* 2010;62(6):929.e1-929.e9.

150. Hirshkowitz M. National sleep foundation's sleep time duration recommendations: Methodology and results summary. *Journal of National Sleep Foundation.* 2015:40-43.

151. Sherwood L. *Human physiology: From cells to systems.* second ed. United States of America: West Publishing Company; 1989.

152. Buman MP, Kline CE, Youngstedt SD, Phillips B, Tulio de Mello M, Hirshkowitz M. Sitting and television viewing: Novel risk factors for sleep disturbance and apnea risk? results from the 2013 national sleep foundation sleep in america poll. *Chest.* 2015;147(3):728-734.

153. Lindseth G, Lindseth P, Thompson M. Nutritional effects on sleep. *West J Nurs Res*. 2013;35(4):497-513.

154. Buman MP, Phillips BA, Youngstedt SD, Kline CE, Hirshkowitz M. Does nighttime exercise really disturb sleep? results from the 2013 national sleep foundation sleep in america poll. *Sleep Med*. 2014;15(7):755-761.

155. Crum AJ, Corbin WR, Brownell KD, Salovey P. Mind over milkshakes: Mindsets, not just nutrients, determine ghrelin response. *Health Psychol*. 2011;30(4):424-9; discussion 430-1.

156. Crum AJ, Langer EJ. Mind-set matters: Exercise and the placebo effect. *Psychol Sci*. 2007;18(2):165-171.

157. Brown B. *Daring greatly.* New York, New York: Penguin Group; 2012.

158. Peters J, Parletta N, Lynch J, Campbell K. A comparison of parental views of their pre-school children's 'healthy' versus 'unhealthy' diets. A qualitative study. *Appetite*. 2014;76:129-136.

159. Sawka KJ, McCormack GR, Nettel-Aguirre A, Swanson K. Associations between aspects of friendship networks and dietary behavior in youth: Findings from a systematized review. *Eat Behav*. 2015;18:7-15.

160. Greenwood BN, Fleshner M. Exercise, stress resistance, and central serotonergic systems. *Exerc Sport Sci Rev*. 2011;39(3):140-149.

161. Seligman ME. Learned helplessness. *Annu Rev Med*. 1972;23:407-412.

Printed in the United States
By Bookmasters